HEALTH PHYSICS
OPERATIONAL MONITORING

HEALTH PHYSICS
OPERATIONAL MONITORING

Editors
CHARLES A. WILLIS
Potomac Electric Power Co.

JOHN S. HANDLOSER
E. G. & G., Inc.

GORDON AND BREACH, SCIENCE PUBLISHERS
NEW YORK • LONDON • PARIS

Copyright © 1972 GORDON AND BREACH, Science Publishers, Inc.
440 Park Avenue South, New York, N.Y. 10016

Library of Congress Catalog Card Number: 78-188888

Editorial office for Great Britain
    Gordon and Breach, Science Publishers Ltd.
    41-42 William IV Street
    London, W.C. 2, England

Editorial office for France
    Gordon and Breach
    7-9 rue Emile Dubois
    Paris 14e, France

ISBN 0 677 13670 6 (cloth); ISBN 0 677 13675 7 (paper)

Printed in the United States of America

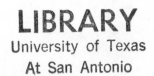

PREFACE

Operational monitoring is the essential part of health physics. While research and the other more esoteric aspects are important, the mainstay of the health physics profession is operational monitoring. The importance of the subject matter combined with the lack of any other comprehensive reference on the subject provides a special impetus for the publication of these transactions.

The principal purposes of this publication are, first, to disseminate applied health physics information; second, to provide a basic reference document for field health physicists; third, to provide a convenient way of introducing the health physics student to operational problems, and finally, to promote the writing of a textbook on applied health physics. While the shortcomings of a symposium-proceedings book are obvious, it is hoped that these volumes will meet the outstanding immediate needs, at least until the long-sought applied health physics text appears.

Partially as a result of the volume of material to be accommodated, the discussions associated with each paper have been omitted. In several ways this is regrettable. Questions and answers are often both interesting and informative. Further, comments might alert the reader and remind him that the various papers represent the views of the authors and not necessarily the position of the health physics profession. For example, Dr. Wegst's comments on the public relations constraints on communications met with objections from Mr. R. L. Kathren. Similarly, Dr. K. Z. Morgan voiced some noteworthy objections to Mr. C. J. Sternhagen's evaluation of uranium mining hazards. There was, in fact, considerable spirted discussion which cannot be included here. It is hoped that these comments will be made available through the journals.

This book and the meeting it reports were made possible by the support of many people. The assistance and encouragement of the Health Physics Society directors, particularly President Langham, were vital. The unflagging efforts of the members and directors of the Southern California Chapter and the committee members in particular, are gratefully acknowledge. This publication, from the selection of the papers through compilation and correction of the proofs, has largely been the responsibility of Mr. John Handloser and the Program Committee. Ultimately, of course, any success enjoyed by this book is due to the contributors.

Charles A. Willis, General Chairman

v

TABLE OF CONTENTS

VOLUME ONE

Session VIII
EDUCATION AND TRAINING

Chairman

RICHARD W. DONELSON
Van Nuys, Calif.

HEALTH PHYSICS EDUCATION AND TRAINING: PAST, PRESENT, AND FUTURE

Roger J. Cloutier*
Oak Ridge Associated Universities, Inc.
Oak Ridge, Tennessee

INTRODUCTION

Before we can relate education and training to
the operational health physicist, we must define
what we mean by an operational health physicist. In
simple terms he is responsible for the day-by-day
radiation safety. He is found in all parts of the radiation industry and can be credited for much of the success the industry has had in achieving its excellent
safety record. The operational health physicist is
frequently called an applied health physicist to dis-
tinguish him from his counterpart, the research
health physicist.

Mr. J. Lenhard has described the operational
health physicist as the person for whom the research
health physicist works. After the research health
physicist establishes basic principles or develops new

---

*Under contract with the United States Atomic
Energy Commission.

instrumentation, the operational health physicist must "... find a way to get the atomic energy business carried out... with reasonable exposures."[1]

To accomplish this task the operational health physicist must not only be knowledgeable but also to work closely with engineers and researchers.

WHAT CONSTITUTES ADEQUATE KNOWLEDGE ?

When I think of radiation safety and education, I am reminded of Dr. Marshall Brucer's[2] statement:

> "Radioisotopes are among the most safe of all materials because it is so easy to detect them. With no other kind of poison is it so easy to determine the approximate location and the approximate strength with so great precision and so little education."

Many of us would agree with this statement but would add quickly that the little knowledge that permits you to know the amount and location of a radioisotope is not adequate for a solution to a radiation safety problem.

On the other hand, Mr. Al Breslin has accused the health physicist of frequently being totally absorbed in the measurement and documentation of the radiation environment and no more than passively interested in the basic design of radiation safety at his facility. If we are to achieve effective and economic health protection, Mr. Breslin feels that the health physicist should play a greater role in the design of ventilation, air cleaning, waste treatment, and similar engineering problems.[3]

At this point, apparently all we need to do is agree on what specific knowledge is required of an operational health physicist and to get on with the task of providing proper education and training. This task is not so simple. Because of the variety in the types of operational health physicists, no single program of training and education would be adequate nor desirable.

The problem is further compounded because operational health physicists are required with a wide range of competence from slightly trained to highly educated with no sharp demarcation between the two groups (Fig. 1). In fact, most professional health physicists occasionally perform technician-level tasks and technicians are sometimes required to perform at a professional level.

What constitutes adequate knowledge? It depends on the responsibility assigned to the operation health physicist.

EDUCATION AND TRAINING

The operational health physicist enters the radiation protection profession at a level based on his ability, experience, and education and training (Fig. 2). By augmenting his ability and experience with further education and training, he is assigned more responsibility. Education and training, therefore, play an important part in the development of the operational health physicist.

We usually think of training and education as being the same. They are not. Training emphasizes imitation while education emphasizes creative interaction.

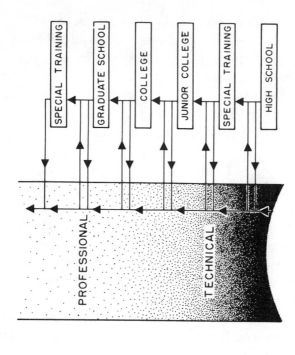

Fig. 1. Distribution of Health Physicists.
The Dots Represent the Relative Number
of Health Physicists at Each Level.

Fig. 2. Routes for Advancement in the
Health Physics Profession.

In general, training emphasizes short-range, limited goals; education emphasizes long-range, broad goals. Training asks "how?" Education asks "how and why?" Training ensures that a person will react in a given way to a given situation. Education does not provide all the answers and requires that a person react in a creative way to unusual situations. A well-qualified operational health physicist must have both education and training.

An operational health physicist's education can be divided into three parts. The largest part is usually the formal education he acquired while attending a school or college. Next in importance is the work-oriented education which he gained from creative evaluation of work experiences. Some individuals, even though lacking formal education, show great ability because of their work-oriented education. The last part of a person's educational background can be called self-education. This includes the self-study that the operational health physicist uses to broaden his education background. It might be designed to improve the individual's technical knowledge or may include the study of how others perform creatively. The broadening of one's education through such books as Applied Imagination[4] or How to Win Friends and Influence People[5] is especially important for the operational health physicist whose work requires him to deal with many different types of people.

Like education, training also contains a formal section. Many introductory courses given in high school and college fall in this category. Next is on-the-job training. When used wisely, this form of training can be very important in a person's development; however, on-the-job training is the hardest to control. Its success depends upon the willingness and attitudes of the trainees and instructors. The third section of a person's training consists of self-training that leads to the acquisition of a skill beyond what is normally required.

Recognizing that the operational health physicist's education and training is made of many parts and that health physicists are required for many different types and levels of responsibility, we shall review some of the existing education and training programs to determine how well they meet the requirements of providing operational health physicists.

ACADEMIC PROGRAMS

1. Graduate Programs

A recent AEC publication lists 261 schools having programs in nuclear-related fields from which operational health physicists might be obtained.[6] Generally, however, professional operational health physicists have participated either in the USAEC[7] or the USPHS[8] health physics graduate programs. Dr. K. Z. Morgan[9,10] has written a complete description of the development of graduate education programs in health physics. Since 1950, almost 1200 students have received assistance under the USAEC fellowship program. The USPHS fellowship program has supported approximately 1200 students for postbaccalaureate studies since 1961.[11] In 1967-68 the USAEC health physics fellowship program was funded with $440,000,[12] the USPHS radiological health program with $2,250,000.[11]

From a beginning of two schools in the fall of
1950, the USAEC fellowship program now includes
18 schools.   Table 1 lists the participating schools
and the distribution of students for 1968-69.   Thirty-
two schools are participating in the USPHS radiological health specialist training programs (Table 2).

In both the USAEC and the USPHS fellowship programs the students must be academically acceptable
to the graduate school they plan to attend. However,
the way the students are selected for each program
differs slightly. In the USAEC fellowship program,
selection is based on a review of the student's background by a board that awards the fellowships for all
schools participating in the program. In the USPHS
fellowship program, approval and award of the fellowship are given by the school at which the students
will attend.

Each school participating in these programs is
free to develop its own curriculum and to establish
requirements for awarding degrees. In recent years,
however, some effort has been devoted to standard-
izing the course of study of the health physics fellowship students. There is general agreement that the
graduate student should become proficient in one of
the basic sciences but he should also participate in an
interdisciplinary program because of the interdisciplinary requirements of health physics.

Early USAEC fellowship programs were geared
to training students within a one- or two-year time
limit. Many of these students earned a Master of
Science degree and immediately started to work as
operational health physicists. The more recent policy
of the fellowship program, which permits students to
continue to the Ph.D. level, has produced fewer

Table 1

USAEC Health Physics Fellowship Program

Participating Institutions	Number of Health Physics Students (1968-1969)
Georgia Institute of Technology	2
Harvard University	2
New York University	2
Purdue University	4
Rutgers, The State University	3
Texas A & M University	1
University of California, Berkeley	9
University of Illinois	4
University of Kansas	4
University of Kentucky	0
University of Michigan	3
University of Minnesota	2
University of Pittsburgh	1
University of Puerto Rico	0
University of Rochester	8
University of Tennessee	10
University of Washington	1
Vanderbilt University	18
Total	74

operational health physicists while increasing the number of research health physicists. This does not mean that Ph.D.'s are not required in operational health physics but rather that many of the individuals responsible for fellowship programs at the universities are research-oriented and the Ph.D. degree is awarded for research; therefore, any candidate for the Ph.D. tends to continue in research activities. This situation is not unusual, for the same problem exists in other professions. Raymond L. Murray in a recent article pointed out that Ph.D. graduates in the nuclear field are so strongly oriented toward research that it is difficult to interest them in practical problems.[13]

Recently when it appeared that the USAEC fellowship program would be changed back to a Master of Science program, in hopes of producing more operational health physicists, the Health Physics Society committee on education and training recommended that the present USAEC fellowship program not be changed. They urged, however, that a separate program be initiated for the training and education of operational health physicists.[14] One should not interpret this action as indicating that the research health physicist is more important than the operational health physicist. Dr. Stannard has often pointed out that neither the operational nor the research health physicist is better than the other—only different. In all fairness students should be stimulated to enter that branch of health physics where they can best perform. The stimulation for operational health physicists might best be provided by operational health physicists working as part-time instructors or consultants for the universities.

Table 2

Schools Participating in Radiological Health
Specialist Training Program

1. University of Arkansas Medical Center, Little
   Rock, Arkansas 72205
2. Auburn University, Auburn, Alabama 36830
3. University of California, Los Angeles, California 90024
4. University of Cincinnati, Cincinnati, Ohio 45229
5. Colorado State University, Fort Collins,
   Colorado 80521
6. Columbia University, New York, New York 10032
7. University of Florida, Gainesville, Florida 32603
8. Georgia Institute of Technology, Atlanta, Georgia
   30332
9. Harvard University, Boston, Massachusetts 02115
10. Iowa State University, Ames, Iowa 50010
11. Johns Hopkins University, Baltimore, Maryland
    21205
12. University of Kansas, Lawrence, Kansas 66044
13. University of Miami, Coral Gables, Florida 33124
14. University of Michigan, Ann Arbor, Michigan
    48104
15. University of Minnesota, Minneapolis, Minnesota
    55455
16. New York University Medical Center, Tuxedo,
    New York 10016
17. University of North Carolina, Chapel Hill,
    North Carolina 27515
18. North Dakota State University, Fargo, North
    Dakota 58103
19. Northwestern University, Evanston, Illinios 60201

Table 2 (Cont'd.)

20. University of Oklahoma, Norman, Oklahoma 73069
21. Oregon State University, Corvallis, Oregon 97331
22. University of Pennsylvania, Philadelphia, Pennsylvania 19140
23. University of Pittsburgh, Pittsburgh, Pennsylvania 15213
24. Purdue University, Lafayetter, Indiana 47904
25. Rensselaer Polytechnic Institute, Troy, New York 12181
26. Rutgers, The State University, New Brunswick, New Jersey 08903
27. Temple University, Philadelphia, Pennsylvania 19140
28. University of Tennessee, Knoxville, Tennessee 37196
29. Texas A & M University, College Station, Texas 77843
30. University of Texas, Austin, Texas 78712
31. University of Washington, Seattle, Washington 98105
32. Yale University School of Medicine, New Haven, Connecticut 06510

One measure of how valuable the fellowship program has been is that 81% of former USAEC health physics fellows are still employed in a nuclear-related profession, Table 3.[12]

Perhaps a better measure of how valuable the fellowship program has been in providing operational health physicists is the number of fellows who become certified by the American Board of Health Physics (ABHP).

Table 3

Employment of Former Health Physics Fellows
1950-51 through 1966-67

	Nuclear	Non-nuclear	Total
Industry	113	28	141
Government	225	14	239
Academic Employment	132	11	143
Military	6	6	12
Further Study	92	17	109
Other	6	56	62
Totals	574	132	706

Most certified health physicists are operational health physicists because the certification examination primarily measures competence in operational health physics. Figure 3 shows the percentage of certified health physicists who had been fellowship students at one of the three major fellowship universities. My alma mater, the University of Rochester, has had the highest percentage of its students becoming certified. This probably can be attributed to an emphasis on operational health physics by the teaching staff at the time the health physicists were fellowship students. Similar data for the USPHS program are not yet available.

2. Undergraduate Programs

Although the education and training of professional health physicists have long been considered a graduate-level program, some effort is now being made to provide programs at the undergraduate level. One of the newest is that funded by the USPHS at the University of Tennessee[15] designed to produce radiation-protection officers. Students entering their junior year with an interest in physics are eligible to enter the program. In addition to the formal course work, students will spend three full quarters in a practicum at Oak Ridge National Laboratory working with the Health Physics Division. At the completion of the course of study, students will be awarded a Bachelor of Science degree in physics with a specialization in the technology of radiation protection.

Of the many universities and colleges having curricula in the nuclear field, specific programs of interest to the operational health physicist include that of the University of Alabama at Birmingham, which offers its physics students a health physics option, and the University of Kansas program in radiation biophysics.

With the goal of supplying health physics technicians, many colleges and technical schools, most with support from the USPHS, have initiated two-year training programs (Table 4). Mr. R. L. Kathren and Mr. D. L. Waite in their paper being presented at this meeting on "Training and Certification of Health Physics Technicians" will discuss the role this training will play in meeting the shortage of trained health physics technicians. The Idaho State University program being conducted in conjunction with the National Reactor Testing site is typical.[16] Its curriculum is given in Appendix A.

Many of the two-year technician-training programs are being conducted at junior colleges. The entry of the junior college in health physics training

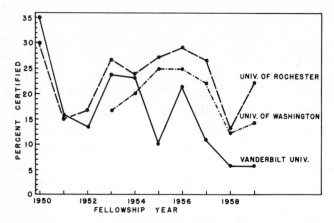

Fig. 3. Percent of USAEC Health Physics
Students Who Have Been Certified by the
ABHP.

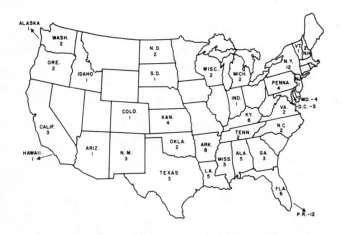

Fig. 4. Distribution of Students Who Have
Attended the ORAU-ORNL 10-Week Health
Physics Course.

Table 4

Colleges Offering Two-Year Training Programs in
Radiation Protection

---

1. Central Florida Junior College, Ocala, Florida
2. Cabot College, Hayward, California
3. Chattanooga State Technical Institute, Chattanooga, Tennessee
4. Columbia Basin College, Pasco, Washington
5. Dobbins Area Vocational Technical School, Philadelphia, Pennsylvania
6. El Camino College, El Camino College, California
7. Hudson Valley Community College, Troy, New York
8. Idaho State University, Pocatello, Idaho
9. Lowell Technological Institute, Lowell, Massachusetts
10. Manhattan College, New York City, New York
11. Montgomery Junior College, Tacoma Park, Maryland
12. Oklahoma State University Technical Institute, Stillwater, Oklahoma
13. Southern Nevada Vocational Technical Center, Las Vegas, Nevada
14. Wentworth Institute, Boston, Massachusetts

---

is especially desirable because the function of the junior college is active dynamic teaching rather than research.

Junior colleges may also serve by providing the large number of operational health physics technicians that will be required at nuclear power plants as the nuclear power industries grow. The health physics technician at a power reactor, however, differs from others in that his health physics duties occupy only part of his time. He is also required to perform water chemistry or other tasks. His training program, therefore, should include practical courses in chemistry, electronics, and industrial safety.

SHORT COURSES

Most operational health physicists have taken a short training course to advance their knowledge. Playing a major role in providing this type of training is the National Center for Radiological Health (NCRH).[17] The center offers the courses listed in Table 5. To conduct these courses the NCRH has a full-time staff of about 30 specialists in radiological health and uses lecturers from other governmental agencies, universities, medicine, and industry. Fourteen training manuals based on more than 400 lectures and laboratory sessions are used in the short-course program.[11]

Another program of short courses is presented by the Special Training Division of Oak Ridge Associated Universities (ORAU) for the USAEC.[18] These courses are designed for users of radioisotopes and other sources of radiation. The objective of these courses is to enable the students (approximately 7000 to date) to use radioactivity in research and industry. Health physics instruction is included in order that the students can safely handle millicurie quantities of radioisotopes. The training students receive in these courses is sufficient to qualify them for an AEC license.

Table 5

National Center for Radiological Health Training
and Manpower Development Program
June 1968 to June 1969

Course Description

Basic Radiological Health
Occupational Radiation Protection
Medical X-ray Protection
Radiological Health for Nurses
Radiological Health for X-ray Technologists
Reactor Safety and Hazards Evaluation
Management of Radiation Accidents
Operational Aspects of Radiation Surveillance
Chemical Analysis of Environmental Radionuclides
Radionuclide Analysis by Gamma Spectroscopy
Measurement of Airborne Radioactivity
Statistical Method-Evaluation and Control for the
    Laboratory
Introduction to Automatic Data Processing Systems

Some courses at ORAU are specifically designed
for training health physicists. The most significant
to the operational health physicist is the 10-week
health physics course for state radiological health
personnel and other eligible persons. Since the first
10-week health physics course in 1962, 115 students
from 35 states (Fig. 4) have been trained. The
course is now offered biannually for approximately
16 students per course. The 400-hr course, conducted
jointly by ORAU-ORNL, is an extremely intensive
training program composed of roughly one half lecture

and one half laboratory (Table 6). The course differs from a university course not only by being intense and relatively short-term but also by including only topics directly related to health physics. Essentially the health physics content of a university health physics program is condensed into 10 weeks and taught from a practical standpoint. Many of the participants of this course have become directors or assistant directors of state regulatory programs.

The ORAU Special Training Division also has conducted several 3-week advanced health physics courses. The advanced health physics course provides structured training in specialized areas of applied health physics.

Specialized health physics training courses for state personnel have been given in various parts of the country by the USAEC Division of State Relations.[19] The courses conducted so far have been on the safe use of medical radioisotopes and industrial radiographic sources.

The USAEC Division of Operational Safety[20] has sponsored a 4-week program on accelerator radiation monitoring and health physics, which was presented at the Lawrence Radiation Laboratory, and also sponsors a 3-day program for physicians who work at a nuclear facility to provide the physician with sufficient information on how to handle a radiation accident.

The National Science Foundation, in conjunction with the USAEC, sponsored a summer institute on health physics for small college radiological safety officers at ORAU in 1967.

Other courses of interest to the operational health physicist include those presented by the Massachusetts Institute of Technology in the summer of 1968 on power

Table 6

Summary of ORAU-ORNL 10-Week Health Physics Course Content

Subjects	Lecture Hours	Laboratory and Field Training Hours	Total
Basic Radiation Physics and Chemistry	33	33	66
Radiation Detection and Measurement	39	48	87
Health Physics Orientation	7	0	7
Radiation Biology and Medicine	19	25	44
Radiation Protection and Control	24	35	59
Administrative Health Physics	8	0	8
Applied Health Physics	19	90	109
Reviews and Exams	20	0	20
Totals	169	231	400

reactor safety,[21] and health physics training programs being presented by private industry.[22,23]

An idea of the number and types of courses on radiation protection that are offered internationally can be gained from the IAEA bimonthly report on conferences, meetings, and training programs in atomic energy.[24]

TRAINING METHODS AND MATERIALS

1. Training Manuals

Most training programs have a manual, consisting of basic atomic and nuclear physics and health physics principles. There are almost as many training manuals as groups conducting programs. Although this duplication of effort is somewhat wasteful, it does have the value that the person preparing the manual receives an education during its preparation. It forces the compiler to examine the basic concepts and to relate them to the group that will use the manual. If he is successful, radiation safety is markedly advanced; if not, he has simply "reinvented the wheel."

Most training manuals resemble textbooks[25-27] and are intended for use in a formal course of study. Others, such as the programmed learning books, are intended for self-instruction. By asking a question or requiring the filling of a blank, programmed learning books introduce a challenge while allowing the student to proceed at his own rate. To be really successful, a programmed learning text must require a student to think and to make judgments. It should reinforce correct answers and point out why a wrong answer is wrong. Two programmed texts on health physics topics have recently been published—Radiation Monitoring[28] and Radiation Safety and Control.[29]

2. Computers

The newest innovation in training and education involves the use of computer-assisted instructions.[30] One advantage of the computer over the programmed learning text is that it can be more versatile. With computer-assisted instruction, the student, while progressing at his own rate of speed, is questioned about a particular fact. If he responds correctly, the next question will be more difficult. But, if he answers incorrectly, he will be questioned on a more basic fact. This question-answer procedure can be conducted in such an order that the student will arrive at the proper answer by logic.

The computer can, in addition, analyze the response of the student and modify the instructional program to match the differences in motivation and ability among students. The computer also provides statistical information to the instructor that is useful in the preparation of the next course of study.

As computer programs on radiation safety become available, we must avoid reinventing the wheel but rather make use of programs already developed. Perhaps the Health Physics Society's committee on education and training could publish a list of available programs once each year.

3. Movies and Television

Movies have played an important part in most health physics training programs. The major producers of radiation safety films have been the USAEC,[31] USPHS,[32] and the armed services.[33] Many of these films are excellent and will remain useful for a long time. Films such as the USAEC's SL-1 Accident will remain of great value for many years and should be included in any session on emergencies. Most films can have greater effectiveness if they are followed by a discussion led by an experienced discussion leader.

In addition to movies, closed-circuit television and videotape recording can be used to advantage in health physics training and education programs. Closed-circuit television permits several students to view procedures that normally can only be viewed by a few students at one time or to view procedures in inaccessible areas such as very high radiation areas.

Videotape may be used to record a lecture and demonstration that must be used over and over to train the same type of group but at different times. These tapes can be used to show methods of operating laboratory equipment, conducting a survey, or removing contaminated clothing. The main advantage of videotape are relatively low cost and the ability to update the tape quickly by editing or re-recording. Much of the basic equipment required for closed-circuit television and videotape recording is already available in many process and power plants.[34,35] It needs only to be adapted to health physics training and education.

Videotape training programs, like movies, should be followed by a discussion period.

The videotape recording system can also be used to assist the health physicist in controlling external radiation exposure. The health physicist has long relied on the control of "time" for the control of exposure.

This is really a time-motion problem. Tapes made with a small, portable camera will permit the operational health physicist to make a careful time-motion study of complex operations and provide him with the information he needs to improve the radiation safety of the operation.

CONTINUING EDUCATION

Continuing education is a method by which individuals offset and overcome technical obsolescence. It may consist of a refresher course or a course specifically designed to present newly acquired information. In the scientific field where the wealth of knowledge is increasing in great steps, this type of program is especially important. The teaching profession has long recognized the need for continuing education and many states require teachers to take continuing education courses to retain their certification.

The Health Physics Society has provided continuing education opportunities in the form of refresher courses at each of its recent annual meetings. The local chapters of the Health Physics Society are also playing a major role in continuing education. Many have established complete refresher courses to assist their members in studying for the ABHP certification exam. The program presented by the East Tennessee Chapter in 1968 is typical (Appendix B).

SOURCES OF INFORMATION

Many groups are ready to serve the operational
health physicist by providing him with information
on specific topics that will help him evaluate radiation hazards and determine adequate solutions. Some
of the most important groups are the specialized information and data centers.[36,37] Centers of special
interest are Nuclear Safety Information Center, Information Center on Internal Exposure, and Radiation
Shielding Information Center. Most information centers maintain computer-stored bibliographies that
can be automatically and rapidly searched by means
of a few "key" words for information on a specific
topic.[38]

In addition to the information centers, the NCRP,
USAEC, USPHS, IAEA, and many others are publishing reports devoted to health physics topics. Appendix C lists a few of the recent publications from each
of these groups that may be of interest to the operational health physicist. Complete listings may be
obtained by writing to the agency. Journals such as
Health Physics, Nuclear Safety, and Radiological
Health Data and Reports are also sources of current
data on radiation safety problems.

SUMMARY

Education and training programs have played a
major role in providing competent operational health
physicists. Many of the programs available before
1964 are classified and described in the IAEA report,
Training in Radiological Protection: Curricula and

Programming.[39] In the United States, the USAEC
and the USPHS fellowship programs have trained most
professional operational health physicists; however,
the recent trend is for these programs to produce research health physicists. The direction can be changed
if operational health physicists actually become involved in academic programs as instructors and by
having academic personnel accept temporary assignments in operational health physics programs.

   The development of two-year academic programs
is recent years promises to provide the professional
operational health physicist with highly trained technicians thus relieving him of much of the professional
but routine work and permitting him to devote more
effort to radiation safety engineering problems.

   As short-course programs improve in quality
and increase in quantity, the operational health physicist will find that they are important to his development. Governmental agencies will probably continue
to play the major role in providing short training
courses, for their skilled teachers and tested training materials and demonstrations have been very effective. These courses are especially needed for
operational health physicists working by themselves
in small operations. The local chapters of the Health
Physics Society can help in the development of operational health physicists by providing more programs
especially devoted to this topic. Regardless of who
puts on the programs they should be made more
widely available by the use of mobile training vans
that travel across the country presenting courses
right at each nuclear industry site.

   We, as operational health physicists, however,
should not expect education and training to improve

without our help. Each operational health physicist must play an active role in the recruitment and development of better qualified health physicists.

ACKNOWLEDGMENTS

The author acknowledges the help of E. Cramer, ORNL; Myron Fair, ORNL; W. Fisher, BNWL; H. Myer, MRC; G. Kyker, ORAU; and A. Dahl, NCRH, for information and ideas.

REFERENCES

1. J. A. Lenhard, Panel Discussion on "Undergraduate Education as Preparation for Graduate Work in Radiation Protection." In: Proceedings for the Conference on Principles of Radiation Protection, August 24-26, 1966 Oak Ridge, Tennessee, U.S. AEC Report CONF-660815, p. 150, 1967.

2. Dr. Marshall Brucer is also well known for his comments on radiation exposure levels, e.g., Vignettes in Nuclear Medicine No. 19, "The Maximum Ridiculous Dose," published by Mallinckrodt/Nuclear, Box 6172, Lambert Field, St. Louis, Missouri 63145.

3. Personal communication with Mr. Al Breslin, 1969.

4. Alexander F. Osborn, Applied Imagination: Principles and Procedures of Creative Thinking, New York, Charles Scribner & Sons, 1953.

5. Dale Carnegie, How to Win Friends and Influence People, New York, Simon and Schuster, Inc., 1936.

6. Educational Programs and Facilities in Nuclear Science and Engineering, 4th edition, compiled by Special Projects Office, Oak Ridge Associated Universities, Oak Ridge, Tennessee, September, 1968.

7. For information on USAEC health physics fellowships, write Fellowship Office, Oak Ridge Associated Universities, P. O. Box 117, Oak Ridge, Tennessee 37830.

8. For information on USPHS radiological health fellowships, write Arve H. Dahl, Chief, Training and Manpower Development Program, Bureau of Radiological Health, 12720 Twinbrook Parkway, Rockville, Maryland 20852.

9. Karl Z. Morgan, Graduate Programs for the Health Physicist in the United States, Health Physics 11, 895-915, 1965.

10. K. Z. Morgan and J. E. Turner, editors, Principles of Radiation Protection, New York, John Wiley & Sons, Inc., 1967.

11. Arve H. Dahl, National Center for Radiological Health Training and Manpower Development Program, presented at the American College of Radiology, 44th Annual Meeting, Feb. 6-10, 1968, Chicago, Illinois.

12. Personal communication with ORAU fellowship Office, January, 1969.

13. Raymond L. Murray, Nuclear Engineering and the Goals Report, Nuclear News 11, No. 6, 30-33, June 1968.

14. J. N. Stannard and John R. Horan, Comment on the Future of the AEC Speical Fellowship Program, Health Physics 13, 647-648, 1967.

15. For information on the University of Tennessee specialization in radiation protection, write the Physics Department, University of Tennessee, Knoxville, Tennessee.

16. J. W. McCaslin, Health Physics Technician Training, Health Physics 13, 652-654, 1967.

17. For information on the NCRH short courses, write Chief, Health Training Section, National Center for Radiological Health, Rockville, Maryland 20852.

18. For information on courses conducted by ORAU, write Special Training Division, Oak Ridge Associated Universities, P.O. Box 117, Oak Ridge, Tennessee 37830.

19. For information on courses sponsored by USAEC Division of State and Licensee Relations, write Division of State and Licensee Relations, U.S. Atomic Energy Commission, Washington, D.C. 20545.

20. For information on courses sponsored by USAEC Division of Operational Safety, write Division of Operational Safety, U.S. Atomic Energy Commission, Washington, D.C. 20545.

21. For information, write Director of Summer Session, Massachusetts Institute of Technology, Cambridge, Massachusetts.

22. Management Newsletter, Where to Send Your Employees for Nuclear Training: Part I. Electrical World, Vol. 170, No. 19, 49-52, November 4, 1968.

23. Management Newsletter, Where to Send Your Employees for Nuclear Training: Part II. Electrical World, Vol. 170, No. 20, 61-64, November 11, 1968.

24. Conferences, Meetings, Training Courses in Atomic Energy, a list published every two months, IAEA. Vienna, International Atomic Energy Agency.

25. H. W. Stroschein and P. H. Maeser, editors, Health Physics Technician Training Manual, National Reactor Testing Station, U.S. AEC Report IDO-17182, June 1966.

26. Basic Radiological Safety Training Manual, Reynolds Electrical and Engineering Co., Inc., Radiological Safety Division, U.S. AEC Report TID-17025, 1962.

27. H. J. Moe, S. R. Lasuk, and M. C. Schumacher, Radiation Safety Technician Training Course, Argonne National Laboratory, U.S. AEC Report ANL-7291, 1966.

28. James E. Wade and G. E. Cunningham, Radiation Monitoring, a programmed instruction book, U. S. Atomic Energy Commission, Division of Technical Information, Oak Ridge, Tennessee, August, 1967.

29. R. A. Costner, Jr., E. N. Cramer, and R. L. Scott, Jr., Reactor Operator Study Handbook (Programmed Instruction Version), Vol. II, Radiation Safety and Control, U.S. AEC Report ORNL-TM-2034, January 1968.

30. R. C. Atkinson and H. A. Wilson, Computer-assisted Instruction, Science 162, 73-77, 4 October 1968.

31. U. S. Atomic Energy Commission 16 mm Film Catalogs, available from Division of Technical Information, U. S. Atomic Energy Commission, Oak Ridge, Tennessee 37830, request listing for Popular Level or Professional Level.

32. Public Health Service Film Catalog, U.S. Department of Health, Education, and Welfare, Public

Health Service, Washington, D.C., published
annually. (Public Health Service Publication No.
776).

33. Film Reference Guide for Medicine and Allied
Sciences, published annually by the U.S. Depart-
ment of Health, Education, and Welfare, Public
Health Service, Washington, D.C. (Public Health
Service Publication No. 487).

34. J. W. Wheeler, CCTV for Modern Power Plants,
Power Engineering, Vol. 72, No. 9, 49-51, September, 1968.

35. R. L. Moore, Closed-circuit Television Viewing
in Maintenance of Radioactive Systems at ORNL,
U.S. AEC Report ORNL-TM-2032, November
1967.

36. Directory of USAEC Specialized information and
Data Centers, U.S. Atomic Energy Commission,
Division of Technical Information, Oak Ridge,
Tennessee 37830, May 1967.

37. Anthony T. Kruzas, editor, Directory of Special
Libraries and Information Centers, 2nd edition,
Detroit, Gale Research Co., 1968.

38. J. R. Buchanan and Wm. B. Cottrell, A Summary
of NSIC Activities, 1963-1967, U.S. AEC Report
ORNL-NSIC-46, September 1968.

39. International Atomic Energy Agency, Technical
Reports Series No. 31, Training in Radiological
Protection: Curricula and Programming. Vienna,
International Atomic Energy Agency, 1964. STI/
DOC/10/31.

APPENDIX A

Table 1

The Idaho State University Curriculum

Curriculum	First Year	Credits	
		1st Semester	2nd Semester
Biology 107	(Introduction to biology)	4	
CE 101	(Drawing)		2
CE 109	(AEC Orientation)		1
Chemistry 121	(General)	5	
English 101-102	(Composition)	3	3
Mathematics 117-112	(thru Calculus)	5	5
Speech 101	(Principles)		2
Elective			3
		17	17

Second Year

Course		I	II
EE 211	(Circuits)	3	
English 310	(Technical reports)		3
Gen. Business 310	(Human relations)		3
Mathematics 251	(Probabilities)	3	
ME 223	(Materials and processes)	4	
Phys. Educ.		1	1
Physics 211-212	(General)	4	4
Electives			
		15	15

Recommended Electives
CE 207   (Statics)
Other Sciences

Reproduced from Health Physics 13, 652-654, 1967, by permission of the author and the Health Physics Society.

Table 2

NRTS HP Technical Training

Subject	Clock hours
Course introductions	3 1/2
Health and safety indoctrinations	13
Nuclear industry history	2
Library usage	5
Introduction to radiation fundamentals	6
Origins of health physics	3
Health physics organizations	2
Basic physics	18
Radiation dose and dose guides	7
Radiation detection instrumentation	43
Introduction to atomic and nuclear physics	39
Introduction to practical problems	4
Protection from external dose	3
Radioactive contamination control	9
Decontamination	4 1/2
Radioactive waste disposal	8 1/2
Biological effects of radiation	9
Principles of nuclear reactors	4 1/2
X-ray principles	3
Environmental monitoring	9
Transportation of radioactivity	7
Criticality for technicians	3 1/2
Emergency action	8
Spectrometer use	28 1/2
In-plant training and familiarization	269
Special problems, all plants	42
Air monitor chart analyzes	8
Ra-Th problems	6

Table 2 (Cont'd.)

Laboratory and plant tours	35
Seminars	76
Study time	191
Visiting lecturers	12
First aid	20
Laser safety	3
Fire and radiation safety	8
Ventilation and radiation safety	8
Other safety considerations	7
Meteorology and health physics	2
Maintenance problems	2
Training personnel in radiation safety	4
Review	12
Course critique and termination	8
Total	953

APPENDIX B

East Tennessee Chapter of the Health Physics Society
1968 Health Physics ABHP
Certification Training Program

Session No. *	Topics
1	Review of mathematics and physics
2	Atomic and nuclear physics Modes of decay - x rays - background
3	Radioactive decay rates Specific activity and statistics
4	Interaction of radiation with matter - alpha, beta, gamma, and neutron
5	Radiation units
6	Radiation protection limits ICRP, NCRP, FRC, AEC
7	Shielding - x rays, beta, gamma neutron
8	External dosimetry: theory, instruments, mixed fields, personnel
9	Air and water sampling
10	Internal dosimetry - calculation

*Each session two hours long

APPENDIX B (Cont'd.)

11	Bioassay techniques and whole body counting
12	Criticality, reactors, and re-processing
13	X-ray protection
14	Medical uses of radiation
15	Accelerator safety
16	Waste disposal
17	Radiation biology - acute exposure - somatic
18	Radiation biology - chronic exposure - somatic and genetic
19	Laboratory design
20	Radiation accidents - respiratory protection - civil defense

APPENDIX C

Publications on Health Physics Topics

IAEA

1. International Atomic Energy Agency. Safety Series No. 2. Safe handling of radioisotopes; health physics addendum, by G. J. Appleton and P. N. Krishnamoorthy. Vienna, International Atomic Energy Agency, 1960.

2. International Atomic Energy Agency. Technical Reports Series No. 83. Economics in managing radioactive wastes. STI/DOC/10/83. Vienna, International Atomic Energy Agency, 1968.

3. International Atomic Energy Agency. Safety Series No. 21. Risk evaluation for protection of the public in radiation accidents. Vienna, International Atomic Energy Agency, 1967.

4. International Atomic Energy Agency. Technical Reports Series No. 37. Manual for the operation of research reactors. Vienna, International Atomic Energy Agency, 1965. STI/DOC/10/37.

NCRP

1. National Committee on Radiation Protection and Measurements. Safe handling of radioactive materials. Recommendations of the National Committee on Radiation Protection. U.S. Department of Commerce, Washington, D.C., 1964. (NCRP Report No. 30; National Bureau of Standards Handbook 92).

2. National Council on Radiation Protection and Measurements. NCRP Report No. 32. Radiation protection in educational institutions. Recommendations of the National Council on Radiation Protection and Measurements. NCRP, Washington, D.C., 1966.

USPHS

1. Routine surveillance of radioactivity around nuclear facilities, December 1966. Interlaboratory Technical Advisory Committee Report No. 1. U. S. Public Health Service, Washington, D. C., 1967. Environmental Health Series. Radiolobical Health. (PHS Publication No. 999-RH-23).

2. U. S. Department of Health, Education, and Welfare. Particle accelerator safety manual, prepared by William M. Brobeck and associates. U. S. Department of Health, Education, and Welfare, Environmental Control Administration, National Center for Radiological Health, Rockville, Maryland, Medical and Occupational Radiation Program Report MORP 68-12, October, 1968.

3. Reduction of Radiation Exposure in Nuclear Medicine, Proceedings of a symposium held at the Kellogg Center for Continuing Education, East Lansing, Michigan, August 7-9, 1967. U. S. Public Health Service, National Center for Radiological Health, Rockville, Maryland, 1967. Environmental Health Series. Radiological Health. (PHS Publication No. 999-RH-30).

USAEC

1. Eugene L. Saenger, M.C., editor, Medical aspects of radiation accidents, a handbook for physicians, health physicists, and industrial hygienists, U. S. Atomic Energy Commission, Washington, D. C., 1963.

2. J. J. Fitzgerald, G. L. Brownell, and F. J. Mahoney, Mathematical theory of radiation dosimetry, (prepared under the auspices of the U. S. Atomic Energy Commission). New York, Gordon and Breach, 1967.

A STUDY OF THE EDUCATIONAL AND CAREER OPPORTUNITIES FOR RADIOLOGICAL HEALTH TECHNICIANS

Herbert J. Deigl
Cornell University
Ithaca, New York

A person chooses the field of health physics not out of curiosity, but of interest. This field is chosen for a career because it is economically rewarding and is part of a challenging new technology.

In investigating opportunities in Health Physics, our interest was in what the opportunities were for a career in health physics; not why individuals chose that field for a career nor because of the financial benefits which accrued. In exploring the opportunity of such a career, how is motivation initiated in a potential student?

The logical place to start was at the secondary level of our schools. How does a student evaluate and choose career opportunities? It was determined that early contact was made with guidance counsellors. This group is most influential in helping prospective students choose a career. We learned from interviews with guidance counsellors that they were not

well informed about a career in health physics. It
was noted that guidance counsellors were knowledgeable in the more customary technical disciplines.

The geographic location of both student and prospective school, as well as the economic status of his
family are also determining factors in decisions
forming a young person's career goals.

It is apparent that when the doors to a four year
institution are closed, economically and/or scholas-
tically, the student is eager to satisfy his desire for
a higher education through less costly technological
or two year college programs. In many cases this is
a stepping stone to a four year institution. Interaction
is desirable among the students, their school contacts
(the guidance counsellor) and the prospective institutions of higher education.

The geographical location may prevent him from
entering schools of his choice. Consider that the
student does not have a nearby school available that
offers his first choice of curriculum. He will then
settle for his second or even third choice just to fulfill the urge and desire to attend a convenient and acceptable school.

The availability of scholarships to help him economically and the consideration of financial burdens
placed on his family often are determining factors in
seeking a school as close to home as possible. Thus,
he adapts himself to a curriculum offered even though
it is not his direct choice.

The student's attitude toward securing a position
upon high school graduation has changed in the past
ten or twelve years. He now realizes that the opportunity for a position is much better if he has advanced training with an associate degree. He is

desirous of graduating because of the opportunities
awaiting him.

Two year colleges draw students from approximately a 125 mile radius. Upon graduation, they
generally remain in this area. Radiation Health,
Health Physics, Nuclear Technology are being offered
as special fields in these programs.

Four years ago it was almost impossible to study
graduates of Junior Colleges that offered a degree in
these fields. I first investigated the northeastern
states north from Washington, D. C., and east from
Ohio. In this area there were less than ten associate
degree students to follow.

Today 7 schools have curriculums in Radiation
Controls in their programs. (Table I).

More emphasis on communication and interaction
with students attending secondary school now, through
their guidance counsellors, is required by the Junior
Colleges and technological schools. Many stimulating
opportunistic positions are available and waiting to be
filled. It is also the responsibility of the Health Physics Society to communicate with educators and students.

We should envision this student as a graduate of
a two year college. He will, upon graduating, be able
to assist any health physicist with the least amount
of on-the-job training. He will be valuable because of
his diversified and specialized academic background.
He will know the "whys" as well as the "hows".

Let us now pose several questions for consideration. First, is preparation for practice in this field
one that can be effectively taught in a college? If so,
is the community college the appropriate institution?
Second, what skills, knowledge and attitudes must be
taught to enable the graduate to function successfully

Table I

Community (Junior) Colleges Surveyed

COLLEGE	Length	Day or Evening	Degree
Central Florida Junior College	2 years	Day	Associate
Dobbins Institute of Technology	1½ years	Day	Certificate
Lowell Institute of Technology	5 years	Evening	Associate
Oklahoma Technological Institute	2 years	Day	Associate
Montgomery County Junior College	2 years	Both	Associate
Hudson Valley Community College	2 years	Day	Associate
Manhattan College	3 years	Evening	Certificate

in this field? Third, what kinds of formal education, work experience, and preparation for teaching are presently utilized, and what alternatives will best prepare an instructor in this field? Fourth, is the field presently ready to set educational standards, or accept existing standards of professional organizations? If so, what are the standards?[1]

To try to answer these questions, information was needed on prospective areas of employment open to the graduates of two year community colleges, as well as the colleges themselves. In order to acquire this information, a questionnaire was sent to prospective employers in over 150 nuclear facilities. The covering letter sent with the questionnaire described the need for the survey and spelled out the roll of the technician. It was rather successful for only in one instance was the title Radiation Control Technician spoken of not fully understood.

Classifications were:

I University Hospitals

II Manufacturing, including Nuclear Power
   Reactors

III State, Health Departments and Government
   Service

IV Isotope Production

V Irradiation Services, Universities and Instrument Manufacturers and others

In order to get a fairly representative cross-
section of the nuclear industry, it was decided to poll
the above categories. Equal value was given each
completed questionnaire regardless of the size of the
facility or the number of people employed.

Approximately 43 per cent of the questionnaires
were returned out of 166. Of this total 77 per cent
replied that they employ Radiation Control Technicians;
23 per cent replied that they do not hire Radiation Control Technicians. Despite the use of the title "Radiation Health Technician" in the questionnaire, it was
noticed that the range of job code classifications used
in the answers was seemingly endless.

It is interesting to note that among a selection of
297 specific occupation categories of those in which
at least 500 persons were employed in the health service industry, there was no mention of Radiation Controls Technician.[2] University hospitals may include
such titles as Laboratory Assistant, Film Badge
Technician, Radioisotope Technologist and Radiological Safety Specialist. Manufacturers, States, Government Service, Isotope Producers and other services

use titles such as Radiological Control Officer, Public Health Physicist Technician, Health and Safety Technician and Technical Aides. In all, over 20 individual titles were used most of which are not listed in generally used lists of occupational titles.

Titles used do not in every instance denote exactly the technician's prime role. If, in fact, it is one of control and safety, then but a few convey this. In many cases the question asking for the title of job code classification for the Radiation Control Technicians was left blank. Thus, no statistical count could be made because of an inexact description of title.

Many technicians are hired with little or no experience. Our survey showed that 23 out of 48, or 48 per cent, had no previous experience. All underwent some form of on-the-job training after being hired. Three students (16 per cent) of the 19 Associate Degree employees were graduates of two year radiological degree programs. Because of the relatively few students with associate degrees in Radiation Controls, the remaining two year students, it would seem, are from technical schools. (Table II).

Because of the relatively few graduates, most of the data is based on returns from employers. However it is interesting to note that in the seven schools under study a total of 142 technicians have graduated to date. (Table II).

Twenty-five questionnaires were sent to technicians who had been surveyed three years ago as students. The question eliciting information on their job descriptions had some rather surprising results. (Table III).

Table II

Status of Schools as of 12-68

COLLEGE	Enrolled to date	Graduated to date	Expect to graduate June 1969
Central Florida Junior College	42	20	10
Dobbins Institute of Technology	18	12	2
Lowell Institute of Technology	75	0	8
Oklahoma Technological Institute	123	42	15
Montgomery County Junior College	65	11	13
Hudson Valley Community College	63	30	10
Manhattan College	92	27	10
	478	142	68

Table III

Follow up study of 25 technicians with Associate Degrees

in RadHealth

Number	Occupation
2	In service
2	Chemical Technicians
3	Radiological Control Technicians
8	Students, 4 year institutes
2	Environmental Technicians
8	No answer

This might indicate that although the schools are graduating students, not all of them are pursuing a career in health physics.

The relatively small number of returns might at first appear not significant. However when one looks at the number of graduates to date, 142, you see that this represents 16 per cent. Also it must be emphasized that these graduates were the earliest in the program. At this time there were less than 50 student graduates.

There seems to be no specific ladder to success and the normal attributes associated with successful technicians apply to the group we are studying. Most employers agree that extra academic training is essential for promotion. If the worker is associated with a union then the ingrade raises seem to be automatic. The promotions a man gets are based on merit. Some facilities give both oral and written examinations to determine the qualifications for promotions.

The general across-the-board annual or semi-annual raises range from 5 to 8 per cent. Concern was shown with the pay scale in some areas—Radiation Health being one of them, as being too low and making the hiring of a two-year degree man almost impossible. The five groups are fairly consistent in salary. Table IV gives the groups and the average salaries. It would appear that manufacturing is again in the lead. The minimum salary for the manufacturing group is some $300.00 above the mean starting average for all groups. The top salary is almost $1400.00 above the mean top salary. The salary scale in government service is slightly less but still more than the fifth group that includes irradiation

services, universities and instrument manufacturers.
Salaries in isotope production are very close to the
mean average.

Table IV

Average yearly salary all groups.

Group	Classification	Salary Starting	Top
I	University Hospitals	$ 6060 -	7780
II	Manufacturing, including Power Reactors	5579 -	8700
III	State, Health Departments Federal Government	4985 -	6925
IV	Isotope Production	5383 -	7033
V	Services, Universities, Instrument Manufacturers, Others	4476 -	6333
	Mean Average	5297 -	7354

The above salaries have been reduced to per
annum and no distinction is made between hourly paid
employees and salaried employees.

In trying to upgrade the classification of the Radiation Control Technicians we should strive to obtain the majority of our technicians from two-year
colleges. In order to secure the best technicians the
society should formulate a program of educating the
guidance counsellors in secondary schools in the
need for Radiation Control Technicians. It should
also inform the general public and remove forever
the stigma of the Mushroom Cloud.

Many times the students are dubious about entering the Radiation Control profession because of a
fear of the consequences of working with radiation
producing isotopes and equipment. For all Atomic

Energy Commission operations in 1964 there was
1.96 average number of disabling injuries per each
million employee hours worked, compared with an
average of 12.3 for all manufacturing industries.[3]

It should be the primary responsibility of this
society to supply the guidance counsellors with the
necessary tools so that they may be more able to
guide students toward a career in health physics.
It must be the duty of the Health Physics Society to
formulate a need for standards for the Radiation Control Technician. We should make these standards
applicable to a technician who might work in a hospital
as a radioisotope specialist as well as a technician
who desires work in a reactor facility. We must be
sure to include all areas of employment so that the
high school student knows he has many opportunities
to choose from.

We should be able to educate technicians who are
not limited to rote gained knowledge. We have been
functioning as a unit for many years and it is time
that we did something to make available technicians
of the highest calibre.

The Health Physics Society should be a leader
in instigating a firm policy not only to set standards
for technicians but to define the duties and confirm
the title of Radiation Control Technician.

It should be the aim of this society to adopt a
standard title to describe in a few words the role of
the Radiation Technician in Safety Control in the nuclear industry. It is my belief that Radiation Control
Technician is such a descriptive title. We should,
at the same time, be looking in the future to the day
that these technicians will be certified. Our society
should set the standards for such a certification

program. With the title clearly defined, we must then standardize the levels of professionalization and upgrade them for future trends.

REFERENCES

1. R. E. Kinsinger and M. Ratner. Technicians for the Health Field: A Community College Health Careers Study Program. University of the State of New York.

2. Dictionary of Occupational Titles, U. S. Employment Service, U. S. Government Printing Office, 3rd ed. , 1965.

3. Occupational Outlook.Handbook, U. S. Department of Labor, Bulletin No. 1450. 1966-67 Ed.

TRAINING AND CERTIFICATION
OF HEALTH PHYSICS TECHNICIANS*

R. L. Kathren and D. A. Waite**
Battelle Memorial Institute
Pacific Northwest Laboratory
Richland, Washington

ABSTRACT

At least twelve formal programs in radiation monitoring or radiation technology have been established at
the post-high school level, many of which lead to an
associate degree. These programs are described and
compared in light of the needs and functions of the
operational health physics technician. Actual experience with the establishment and operation of two such

*This paper is based on work performed under
United States Atomic Energy Commission Contract
AT(45-1)-1830.

**Technical Institute, Oklahoma State University,
Stillwater, Oklahoma

programs indicates a need for laboratory equipment, instructors with field experience, and support by the nuclear industry, particularly with regard to placement of personnel. To ensure a minimum level of competence among health physics technicians, a certification program patterned along the lines of that maintained by the American Board of Health Physics is proposed, but implemented by a combined board of Certified Health Physicists and health physics technicians.

INTRODUCTION

Throughout science and engineering, professional personnel are assisted by technicians--persons with lesser training who perform myriad tasks in support of the professional. Health physics is no different in this regard. The training and quality control of these technicians is important to the proper conduct of health physics programs. The purpose of this paper is to discuss available training programs at the college level for health physics technicians and to promulgate certification as a means of quality control.

PROGRAMS IN RADIATION TECHNOLOGY

Five years have now elapsed since W. D. Carlson and J. W. Lepak published a study on the needs and curricula for radiological technicians and radiological training.[1] In this time, several types of technician training programs have been instituted and are now in

operation. Some of these programs follow the 1963
recommendations quite closely while others have
adopted little from the report. A summary of the resulting diversity of curricula now available is illustrated in Table I.

Twelve colleges are known to have programs now,
with one in the final stages of development. All programs are essentially on the community (junior) college level. Even though the graduates of these programs will likely be employed under similar job
titles with similar job responsibilities, it is obvious
from the data that these similarities are not at all
based on equality of preparation and background in
the fundamentals of radiation technology. Although
on-the-job training receives varying degrees of emphasis in the different curricula, according to the different program objectives, a preliminary comparison
of some validity can nonetheless be made on the basis
of course distribution.

Categorization of courses which make up the various curricula was made on the basis of radiation monitor preparation needs, utilizing course titles and catalog descriptions. Of necessity, variations in the quality of the actual offering were not considered. Courses
considered fundamental to the future health physics
technician—for example radiation physics, nuclear
technology, radiation health, and radiation biology—
were classified as specialty courses. Courses such
as metallurgy, which might seemingly be placed under
the specialty category for a Nuclear Engineering Technician, were classed as related technical, along with
fundamental electronics, general chemistry, etc. All
non-technical courses were placed in the general
course column.

TABLE I.

SUMMARY OF TECHNICIAN TRAINING PROGRAMS

Semester Hours

College	Curriculum Title	Duration*	Total	Specialty	Related Tech.	Gen. Education	On-The-Job Training	Degree*	Comments
Central Florida	Radiolog. Health Tech.	2 Yrs., S	72	26	34	12		A.A.	Includes summer session
Chabot	Radiation Technol.	2 Yrs. (eve),Q	21.3	13.3	4	4		Cert.	In Engr. Div.
Columbia Basin	Radiolog. Technol.	2 Yrs. (eve),Q	23	14	7	2	Implied but not part of curr.	Cert	Monitor upgrading
Dobbins Vocational	Radiolog. Health Technol.	2 Yrs.,S	N.A.*	20	9	3	1 semester full time work		Heavy public health emphasis
Hudson	Public Health Tech.	2 Yrs.,Q	75.3	19.3	43.3	12.7		A.A.S.	Radiolog. Health option
Idaho State U.	Health Physic. Tech.	2 Yrs.,S	64	1	47	16	24 wks	Cert.	761 clock hrs. given in spec. during summer field training
Lowell	Radiolog. Health Technol.	5 Yrs. (eve)	90	33	48	9		A.S.	
Manhattan	Rad. Health & Science	2 Yrs.(eve)T 2 Yrs, T	36 66	21 21	15 15	0 30		Cert. A.A.S.	In Physics Department
Montgomery	Radiol. Science	2 Yrs.,S	65	16	26	23		A.A.	
Nevada So. U.	Radiation Health Technol.	2 Yrs.,S	65	27	25	13		A.S.	In final development stages
Oklahoma State U.	Radiation & Nuclear Tech.	2 Yrs.,S	68	35	23	10	Elective in curr.	A.S.	
Wentworth	Nuclear	2 Yrs,S	80	16	54	10		A. Eng.	Plus non-credit Summer reading course.

* Abbreviation Code
Q, Quarter; S, Semester; T, Trimester; A.A., Associate in Arts; Cert., Certificate; A.A.S., Associate in Applied Science; A.S. Associate in Science; A. Eng. Associate in Engineering; N.A., Not Available.

Of the twelve colleges known to have programs, eight offer a full-time two-year curriculum (or equivalent) leading in all but one case to an associate degree. Five offer certificates of completion for shorter programs that are roughly the equivalent of two-thirds of an academic year. At least one school offers both a certificate and degree program, and others plan to do likewise.

Total semester hours of these curricula vary from 21.3 to 90, with associate degree programs containing more than the Certificate programs, as might be expected. Distribution of courses among the general, support and specialty categories is similarly diverse. Specialty courses command from 20 percent to 62.6 percent of total course time, with certificate programs having a greater ratio than associate degree programs. Specialty and related technical courses constitute from 81.3 to 91.3 percent of the sample curricula, leaving about 15 percent on the average for general education considerations.

The geographical distribution of these schools is interesting, particularly when viewed in relation to major nuclear sites and operating reactors. As seen in Fig. 1, nuclear sites are fairly well distributed geographically. However, with a single exception, only in the West are colleges with programs in proximity to major nuclear centers. This proximity is advantageous in that personnel actively engaged in the nuclear field can be utilized as part of the instructional staff, as part of a symbiotic relationship between the site and the school. Moreover, the community is aware of the nuclear field, and prospective students can foresee local employment at the completion of their training. There are also some disadvantages to proximity,

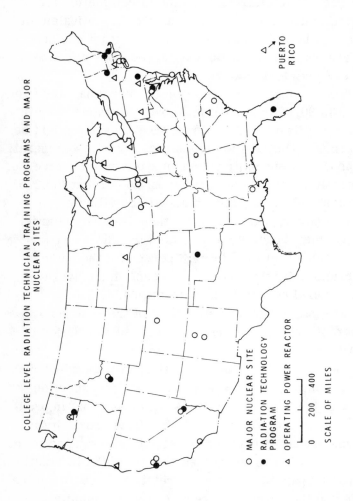

COLLEGE LEVEL RADIATION TECHNICIAN TRAINING PROGRAMS AND MAJOR NUCLEAR SITES

○ MAJOR NUCLEAR SITE
● RADIATION TECHNOLOGY PROGRAM
△ OPERATING POWER REACTOR

SCALE OF MILES

0   200   400

PUERTO RICO

Figure 1

not the least of which may be dependence of the school on the nuclear site, with an undue emphasis on the subject matter and techniques considered important by the local nuclear site.

In addition to the four western schools, only Montgomery, located in the greater Washington, D. C., area, is close to a concentration of organizations that might utilize the services of health physics technicians or persons with training in radiation technology. Nearby are the U. S. Public Health Service National Center for Radiological Health, Atomic Energy Commission Headquarters, the National Bureau of Standards, and the Armed Forces Radiobiology Research Institute.

Of the remaining seven programs, none is proximal to a major nuclear site. Five are localized in the populous Northeast and one in Central Florida. The other program is at Oklahoma State University, and while not close to a major nuclear site, is located in approximately the geographical center of the country As such, it is physically the closest of all programs to at least six major nuclear sites. No programs exist in the populous midwestern states, although within the region are at least three major nuclear sites and six operating reactors with a capacity of nearly 500,000 KWE.

PROGRAM NEEDS

Needs common to most formal radiation technician training programs are students, faculty, equipment and jobs. Major deficiencies in any one of these areas is potentially disastrous to a program. Therefore, it is imperative that institutions offering training progra

exhibit leadership in the valuation and solution of these
needs.

The number of students enrolled in available programs is too small to meet future needs, and in some
cases, to sustain continuous operation of the program.
In part, this is attributable to the relatively small
localized drawing area of most colleges offering these
programs, coupled with a lack of publicity. Since
only about half of the enrollees ultimately graduate,
the large number of dropouts compounds the problem
even more. Much effort is required in this area to
meet projected graduate needs.

Student quality seems to be very good, primarily
because of the enrollment requirements imposed upon
incoming freshmen by most institutions of higher
learning. Quality is further bolstered by significant
numbers of "B" average transfer students from engineering or scientific fields. Some transfers come
from liberal arts curricula, but frequently these students are reluctant to enter such a heavily scientific
and technically oriented area.

Some interesting statistics have been compiled on
a small group of students in several of these programs.[2]
Of the 23 respondents to a questionnaire, five had
prior post-high school education. A personal choice
of radiological health was made by 14, two were influenced by others, but only one of the 23 indicated
that the Guidance Counselor had influenced him.
Three-fourths of the students lived within 20 miles of
the school they were attending, with only one student
being more than 40 miles from home. About half of
the students desired employment within 125 miles of
their homes; none, however, wanted to leave the geographical area in which he was currently located.

This fact is particular interest, when considered with the location of schools in relation to major nuclear sites.

Perhaps the most effective means of boosting these programs is through publicity. Potential enrollees must know of health physics, as must their counselors. An occupational brief entitled "Health Physics Technician"[3] will soon be out in revised form. The lay community must also be educated and informed; certainly there is interest and desire on the part of the public to learn more about nuclear energy.

As proof of this latter contention, the experience of Chabot College can be cited. Located in the San Francisco Bay area, this community college initiated an evening course entitled "Introduction to Nuclear Energy," which had no prerequisites. Announcement of the survey course, which was also designed as the introductory course in a planned radiation technology curriculum, was made in neighborhood newspapers and in the college catalog and schedule of classes. Counselors were made aware of the offering, and helped to acquaint potential students with it.

Approximately 30 students enrolled the first quarter the course was offered. Most (about 75 percent) were not considering a career in the nuclear field and had no previous experience in this area. Many were already established in career patterns—for example, educational backgrounds ranged from high school graduation with a minimum of science and mathematics to a high school science teacher holding a master's degree. Several day students enrolled. Almost all enrolled out of a general interest. Significantly, the attrition rate (about 30 percent) was lower than in most other specialty evening courses at this school

and 12 of those completing the course went on to the
advanced courses. One student was influenced to
major in nuclear engineering at a four year college,
and another entered the nuclear field as a technician.

The success of any program is largely dependent
on its faculty. Full time faculty members are generally young and hold a master's degree in one of the
nuclear fields. However, lack of scientific research
opportunities coupled with a decided lack of field experience and professional participation, often lead
to stagnation, poor knowledge of the field, and low
morale. Excellent opportunities exist for the recti-
fication of these deficiencies through summer industrial placement of teaching faculty. Awareness of
current problems, better utilization of this pool of
available technical manpower, and publishing possibilities are but a few of the potential benefits of such
education—industry cooperative effort. Faculty participation at professional society meeting should also
be encouraged, and funding made available for this
purpose.

Part time faculty members, drawn from the nuclear
field, can supplement the full time faculty. With a
cooperative and active administration, a smaller program could be managed exclusively with part time
faculty members.

Financial restrictions also impose serious limitations on the effectiveness of training curricula. It is
difficult, if not impossible, for a tax-supported technician training program to keep abreast of industry in
terms of equipment. Much of the effort needed to produce a good technician can be wasted with equipment
which is antique by industrial standards and which will
therefore never be used by the technician after graduation.

It is well known that much equipment, more modern than that now possessed by many schools, lies idle within many industrial and governmental laboratories. The maximum utilization of available apparatus should be the concern of the employer as well as of the nuclear industry as a whole. Donation or loan programs could easily be arranged to the mutual benefit of all.

Ultimate success or failure of job-oriented technician training programs depends upon graduate placement. Achievements in this area have been variable and undoubtedly heavily dependent on the approach pursued by both students and administration of specific programs. However, well paying positions are available in quantity to graduates of programs of recognized quality. Student field trips, summer industrial placement of faculty, concentrated student inquiry effort, and confidence are proven means of acquiring industrial cooperation in graduate placement. A summer program of on-the-job training might prove beneficial, both from a training standpoint as well as subsequent job placement.

CERTIFICATION: THE ULTIMATE GOAL

Health physics technicians perform many diverse functions. Many serve as radiation monitors, with heavy responsibilities. Others serve as dosimetry technicians, research assistants, environmental sampling specialists, or in waste disposal and decontamination functions. The importance of the technician within the aggregate health physics program is large, for he serves as the eyes and ears of the professional health physicist. Indeed, the health physics

technician in his role as radiation monitor is often
the only health physics-oriented person with whom
other scientific or technical personnel may deal.

At most of the larger nuclear installations, the
monitor: professional health physicist ratio is in the
neighborhood of 4-5:1. Often, technicians may be
asked to fill the shoes of the health physicist, particularly in emergency situations. Technicians are
also utilized for radiation protection functions in
smaller institutions that cannot justify or afford a
full time health physicist. The relationship of the
technician or monitor to the health physicist is somewhat analogous to that of nurse and physician, with
the nurse serving as both assistant and complement.

Monitors and other health physics technicians
need to be well acquainted with the terminology and
concepts of health physics, as well as the basic
sciences underlying the profession. Because of the
obvious heterogeniety of radiation technician training
coupled with the greatly increasing responsibility delegated to technicians, some mechanism for product
quality control should be devised. This mechanism—
certification—would benefit the training programs
and potential employers as well as the technicians
themselves. The training programs would benefit
from certification through the program evaluation
that would be derived from such a nationwide comparison of graduates. In this manner deficiencies could
be made readily identifiable. There is no such rapid
mechanism presently available to program administrations or funding agencies.

Requirements for certification as a health physics
technician should include some experience and evidence
of familiarity with routine operating problems. To

attempt to spell out an ideal and all-encompassing set
of requirements would be naive; however, the few requirements listed below seem acceptable and work-
able:

1. Course work beyond high school equivalent to
   no less than 60 semester hours of junior or
   technical college level course-work, with at
   least 36 semester hours in the sciences, engineering and radiation technology.

and

2. A minimum of two years of experience in radiation monitoring or other health physics
   technician functions performed in a recognized
   program under the direct supervision of a
   Certified Health Physicist. Additional experience can be substituted for the course work
   described in (1) above on the basis of one year
   for each 15 semester hours.

3. A minimum age of 21 years, and good moral
   character.

4. Recommendation by a Certified Health Physicist or two Certified Health Physics Technicians.

5. Passage of a written examination, as determined by the certifying board.

There would be no grandfather clause; all would take
the examination. Furthermore, it might be well to
close the certification process to those employed as
professional health physicists, and those to whom radiation protection work is secondary.

Certainly there is a precedent for certification of technicians, as exemplified by the certification programs of x-ray technicians and engineering technicians. In the case of both of these groups, uncertified persons can still work in the field, but certification is an important goal that has helped to upgrade both personnel and quality of work.

Potential employers would certainly benefit from the preselection of prospective employees that such a certification program would accomplish. Knowledge that monitors, for example, have evidenced a minimum level of competence is both economically and psychologically reassuring. Management knows too well the price of incompetence.

The benefits of certification to the recipient are well known. Recognition for technical accomplishments, elimination of classification upon the basis of common interest alone, increased salary, job security, and status are but a few. Moreover, the self-satisfaction that accompanies a meaningful certification provides a psychological uplift and increased self-confidence. The resultant evolution of beneficial circumstances would surely follow somewhat the same path as have other such certification programs, both professional and technical, thereby further benefiting those certified as well as the occupational group as a whole.

The major benefactor, however, would be the public. Certification of health physics technicians is decidedly in the public interest if only to ensure a minimum level of competence within a group that daily has the responsibility for human life and well being and thousands of dollars worth of property. Speculate on the consequences of an error directly attributable to

incompetence; the release of curie quantities of radioactivity to the environment, and over-exposure to a
worker that could be disabling or even fatal, or a
criticality accident with a loss of life and tremendous
economic ramifications.

A sound certification program is vital. Such a program could well be moulded along the lines of the professional certification offered by the American Board
of Health Physics. Indeed the ABHP might be the
logical body to administer the program, for it could
then coordinate and relate the certified health physicist. Or perhaps a joint board, either independent
or linked to the ABHP and composed of health physics
technicians and health physicist, could serve as the
certifying body. One point is clear; the operational
health physicist must not abrogate his responsibilities
in the realm of technician certification. He should
actively strive to establish and maintain a dynamic
certification program, providing the leadership and
guidance for which he is uniquely suited. Any meaningful board to certify health physics technicians or
monitors must include representation from the operational health physicist, for without his input, the coin
cannot help but have a hollow ring.

REFERENCES

1. J. W. Lepak, and W. D. Carlson, "Radiological
   Technicians—A Study of the Needs and Recom-
   mended Curricula," University of Nevada Final
   Report for U.S. P. H.S. Contract No. SAph 78542
   (June 14, 1963).

2. H. J. Deigl, Personal communication to D. A. Waite (August 10, 1966).

3. "Health Physics Technician," Chronicle Guidance Publications, 199, 167, (to be published).

IDAHO NUCLEAR CORPORATION
HEALTH PHYSICS TECHNICIAN TRAINING*

H. W. Stroschein, E. A. King,
P. H. Maeser and J. W. McCaslin
Idaho Nuclear Corporation
Idaho Falls, Idaho

ABSTRACT

A two-part program consisting of a classroom
training period and extended formal in-plant is being
conducted by Idaho Nuclear Corporation (IN) to train
health physics technicians for radiation safety control,
Both phases cover operational health physics practices
such as instrumentation usage, radiation and contamination control, safe work permit procedures, and
emergency actions. Training aids include vast physical facilities, two training manuals, an on-the-job
training guide, and extensive instrumentation.

The program is designed to train IN employed
health physics technicians and Idaho State University
Radiation Protection Technology students. The IN
personnel are trained for working in IN operated

---

*Work performed under the auspices of the Atom-
ic Energy Commission

nuclear reactor and radiochemical plant areas while
the Idaho State University sessions are geared to provide broad health physics training to cover the needs
of AEC contractors, universities, laboratories, and
hospitals. The specific requirements and the program variations needed to accomplish training for
each group are discussed.

INTRODUCTION

The demand for trained health physics technicians over the past few years has prompted Idaho
Nuclear Corporation (IN) to conduct a thorough training program for technician trainees. The objective
of the program put succinctly is to train HP technicians for radiation safety control work. The emphasis is upon producing well qualified personnel in a
minimum amount of time. These individuals must
have the ability to recognize potential and existing
radiation hazards in each plant area and advise operational and maintenance personnel in routine situations
involving such hazards. They must also be able to
take or recommend corrective action and perform
first aid in emergency situations until technical health
physics and medical personnel can be summoned.
Technicians with these qualifications have been trained
successfully with a two-part program consisting of a
classroom training period and extended formal in-
plant training.
The program has been developed to train two
groups; (1) IN employee health physics technicians
and (2) students enrolled in the Idaho State University
Radiation Protection Technology Course. The

demonstrated competence of graduates from both groups is indicative of the program's effectiveness. Several individuals thus trained are now in technical health physics positions, in health physics graduate programs, or in responsible positions elsewhere within the nuclear industry. The training for each group will be considered separately.

IN TECHNICIAN CLASSROOM TRAINING

The classroom training period for IN health physics technicians is approximately five weeks depending on the general educational background of the class members. A group that is somewhat deficient in mathematics and/or physics may require a longer classroom training period.

Several thorough reference searches for a satisfactory course text indicated the need for such a publication. A training manual[1] was compiled and released for external distribution. It is used as a nucleus for the classroom training. The manual is "...so arranged that it may be supplemented with specific company policy. The general principles of radiation safety covered include the basic principles of radiation, dose determination and limits, biological effects of radiation, radiation detection instrumentation, contamination control, decontamination, and emergency actions. General information is also included on non-radiological safety often associated with health physics work."[2] Considerable supplementary material is used with this text. A revised edition of the manual is planned for the near future and a portion of this supplementary material probably will be included.

The classroom portion of the IN technician training program is designed to give the technician the
necessary information with a conceptual and practical
approach rather than theoretical.   For instance, in
the discussion of radiation detection instrumentation
the Bragg-Gray Principle is not discussed, nor is
the theory and use of free-air ion chambers.   The
technician is taught such concepts as standard instrument types, what each will detect, its energy de-
pendency, the common operational weaknesses of
each, instrument selection for the job, and meter
reading interpretation.

Exhibit A is a flow chart of a typical course schedule.   The subject material and the order of presentation are the results of a continual review of the program by students, faculty, and management over a ten
year period.   Aphilosophical discussion of the relative time or ordering of each subject will not be covered in this paper.   At least one oral or written exam is given on each area of study.   A passing grade
must be obtained in these exams before credit is giv-
en for satisfactory completion of the course.

Various teaching techniques such as lectures,
demonstrations, supervised use of instruments and
equipment, training films, and programmed teaching
are used in presenting the material.   The degree of
each method used depends upon the number of individuals in each class and their respective and col-
lective backgrounds.   The NRTS library with a motto
of "if we don't have it, we'll get if if it's available"
is an excellent source for reference books, journals,
technical reports, etc., that students might need for
additional information.

Exhibit A

CLASSROOM TRAINING FLOW CHART

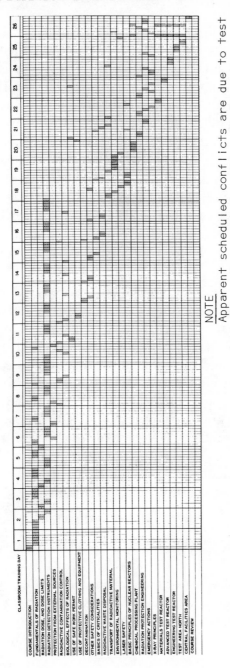

CLASSROOM TRAINING DAY	1	2	3	4	5	6	7	8	9	10	11	12	13	14	15	16	17	18	19	20	21	22	23	24	25	26
COURSE INTRODUCTION																										
FUNDAMENTALS OF RADIATION																										
RADIATION DOSE, AND DOSE LIMITS																										
RADIATION DETECTION INSTRUMENTS																										
PROTECTION FROM EXTERNAL SOURCES																										
RADIOACTIVE CONTAMINATION CONTROL																										
BIOLOGICAL EFFECTS OF RADIATION																										
USE OF SAFE WORK PERMIT																										
USE OF PROTECTIVE CLOTHING AND EQUIPMENT																										
DECONTAMINATION																										
OTHER SAFETY CONSIDERATIONS																										
BASICS OF CRITICALITIES																										
RADIOACTIVE WASTE DISPOSAL																										
TRANSPORT OF RADIOACTIVE MATERIAL																										
ENVIRONMENTAL MONITORING																										
LASER SAFETY																										
BASIC PRINCIPLES OF NUCLEAR REACTORS																										
CHEMICAL PROCESSING PLANT																										
RADIATION PROTECTION ENGINEERING																										
EMERGENCY ACTIONS																										
X-RAY PRINCIPLES																										
MATERIALS TEST REACTOR																										
ADVANCED TEST REACTOR																										
ENGINEERING TEST REACTOR																										
TEST AREA NORTH																										
CENTRAL FACILITIES AREA																										
COURSE REVIEW																										

NOTE

Apparent scheduled conflicts are due to test and review periods of less than one hour.

The philosophy that the course cannot be any better than the teachers teaching it is applied when selecting the faculty. The following qualification guides are used in the selection of instructors: (1) well informed on the subject to be taught, (2) one of the most experienced IN health physics employees on the topic to be taught, (3) desirable attitude toward health physics technician work as a profession, (4) has the desire and personality to teach. The instructors with all of these qualifications have done an outstanding job in the program.

The classroom training for IN technicians also includes a 15 classroom hour Bureau of Mines First Aid course followed by a 2 hour exam conducted by a Bureau of Mines First Aid representative. All IN technicians must complete this course satisfactorily.

Consideration is being given at the present time to a "Learner Controlled Instruction" training program which would reduce the number of classroom class sessions and allow the technician to proceed in the phase of his training at his own speed, thereby allowing him to emphasize the subjects in which he needs training. Instructors will be available for consultation at scheduled times during the training period, but the students' background, need, and ability will dictate his speed of progression.

IN TECHNICIAN IN-PLANT TRAINING

No amount of classroom training can produce an experienced technician. Haphazard experience cannot produce an experienced competent technician effectively or efficiently. Formal, in-plant training supervised by competent, experienced teachers can produce the desired product with a minimum of time and cost.

A good in-plant training program requires plant training facilities and equipment. The following IN contracted NRTS plants are available for training:

1. Three test reactors varying in power output from 40 MW to 250 MW. Refueling and experimental change out shutdowns occur from 3 to 6 weeks apart affording excellent reactor health physics in-plant training.

2. Four pool reactors having power outputs to 1 KW. These reactors are used for criticality studies and reactivity measurements.

3. A chemical processing plant involved in routine fuel reprocessing and fuel reprocessing development. Modular prototypes of many of the future processing techniques are built and tested here. The associated health physics problems provide excellent in-plant training for fuel processing plants of all types.

4. High and low level radiation chemistry labs. These labs provide in-plant health physics training comparable to the needs of most chemistry labs involved in radiation work.

5. A waste calcination facility. This plant provides an excellent training ground for waste management in connection with the chemical processing plant operation.

6. A solid waste burial ground.

7. Four hot cell complexes involving over forty hot cells and caves. High radiation level metalurgy, chemistry and material testing are conducted in these cells and caves. Their associated problems provide excellent health physics in-plant training.

8. A large hot shop where complete reactors are dismantled and their components tested.

9. Extensive decontamination facilities capable of decontaminating large pieces of equipment and small fragile materials, and

10. Three industrial x-ray installations.

Equipment available for training includes:

Numerous gamma spectrometry facilities utilizing scintillation and solid state detection systems, solid state alpha spectrometers, extensive air and water effluent monitoring systems, vast area monitoring complexes, the most modern lab counting equipment available, adequate protective equipment, numerous portable survey instruments for all types of ionizing radiation and two dental x-ray machines set up for instructional purposes.

In addition AEC ID has available bio-analysis labs including whole body counters, film readers, and TLD systems plus extensive waste management and environmental sections.

After completion of the classroom training period each technician trainee is assigned to a specific plant or area. The health physics foreman of that area has the responsibility of all in-plant health physics training. A check list, Exhibit B, is provided as a guide

for the foreman. The foreman can delegate the responsibility of training to a qualified technician. The
individual working with the trainee councils, instructs,
observes, and tests the trainee on each point listed in
the check list. He then initials the check point certifying that the trainee has demonstrated the required
work competence in that subject. It is assumed that
the trainee is not competent to accomplish a specific
task without direct supervision if his check list has
not been initialed for that task. The official training
check list for each IN technician is filed in a training
group center file. It is the responsibility of the
trainee's foreman or the technician delegated by the
foremen to keep this official check list up to date. A
training check list progress report, (Exhibit C) for
the technicians of each area is submitted semi-annually
to the area health physics supervisor and the Health
and Safety Branch manager by the personnel of the
training center.

Upon completion of the green tag (permits to
remove material from radiation control areas),
Safe Work Permit, shipment of radioactive materials, and the non-radiological section of the check
list, the trainee is considered to be a technician.
The non-radiological section consists of industrial
hygiene and safety duties that an IN health physics
technician may have if a plant safety Engineer is
not available. Since the check list includes items
that take lengthy training periods and items that
are peculiar to particular plants, it may take
several years before the technician completes the
entire check list.

IDAHO NUCLEAR CORPORATION

Health Physics Training Check List

Exhibit (B)

Name_____ Date of Hire_____

Assigned Area and period of time (Minimum of 10 consecutive working days)_____

I. Orientation

	Satisfactory Performance Reviewer's Initials	Date
A. Has completed		
1. Health Physics Indoctrination Lecture	_____	_____
2. Safety Indoctrination Lecture	_____	_____
3. Health Physics Course	_____	_____
4. Methods in First Aid Course	_____	_____
5. Familiarization of Personnel Radiation Exposure Records	_____	_____

  B. Has been assigned and adequately tested after studying the following material:

     1. HP Technician Training Manual Chapters
       I. Nuclear History
      II. Birth and Growth of the HP Profession
      III. Organizational Contex
      VII. Radiation, Dose, and Dose Limits
      IX. Protection from External Source of Ionizing Radiation.
      X. Radioactive Contamination Control

	Satisfactory Performance Reviewer's Initials					
	MTR	ETR	ATR	CPP	CFA	TAN
2. Chapter on assigned working area from the "Health Physics Manual of NRTS Areas Operated by IN." (Must have worked in area at least 10 consecutive working days prior to starting on this assignment.)	__	__	__	__	__	__
C. Has been conducted on tour of the working area facility. He is aware of (1) relation of plant layout to function, (2) radiation sources and built-in shielding, (3) contamination sources and contaminants, (4) normal radiation backgrounds in various plant areas. He is familiar with the location of experimental cubicles, storage cells, special laboratories, constant radiation and radioactive contamination monitors, and other plant facilities in the assigned area.	__	__	__	__	__	__

II. Green tag (Form IHP-27) Authorization

A. Has been taught and given duty to make daily routine counter and sensitivity checks and keep records of same.	__	__	__	__	__	__

B. Can operate the following survey instruments
with special attention to differentiating between
different types of radiation.

   1. Cutie Pie   ___ ___ ___ ___ ___ ___

   2. Juno   ___ ___ ___ ___ ___ ___

   3. GM Survey Meter   ___ ___ ___ ___ ___ ___

   4. Alpha Survey Meters   ___ ___ ___ ___ ___ ___

C. Uses proper smear and counting procedures
in a complete contamination check for purpose
of issuing green tags (alpha, beta, gamma).   ___ ___ ___ ___ ___ ___

D. Knows limits allowed for issuance of a green tag.   ___ ___ ___ ___ ___ ___

E. Knows correct procedure for filling out green tag.   ___ ___ ___ ___ ___ ___

F. Has issued at least ten green tags under the supervision of a senior health physics technician.   ___ ___ ___ ___ ___ ___

G. Knows and uses proper procedure for logging
green tag.   ___ ___ ___ ___ ___ ___
At this point the technician should be qualified
to survey for and issue green tags. (Date)   ═ ═ ═ ═ ═ ═

III. Radiation Surveys

A. In addition to instruments listed in II-B
above, has been shown how to operate
and/or has demonstrated proficiency in
operation of: ___ ___ ___ ___ ___ ___

   1. Fast Neutron Survey Meters   ___ ___ ___ ___ ___ ___

   2. Thermal Neutron Survey Meters   ___ ___ ___ ___ ___ ___

B. Has been instructed and shown proficiency in:

   1. Proper selection and testing of survey
instruments.   ___ ___ ___ ___ ___ ___

   2. Proper selection of other necessary
equipment such as radiation tags, ra-
diation ribbons, and marking pencils.   ___ ___ ___ ___ ___ ___

C. Has used instruments and equipment properly in making at least ten beta-gamma
radiation surveys.   ___ ___ ___ ___ ___ ___

D. Has made at least two fast neutron and
two thermal neutron surveys properly and
calculated dose rates correctly.   ___ ___ ___ ___ ___ ___

E. Notifies area supervisor if hazardous
sources are discovered.   ___ ___ ___ ___ ___ ___

F. Properly enters survey results in HP log.   ___ ___ ___ ___ ___ ___

IV. Contamination Survey

Has performed at least ten contamination surveys under the direction of a senior technician.
Specific attention is to be given to:

	Satisfactory Performance					
	Reviewer's Initials					
	MTR	ETR	ATR	CPP	CFA	TAN

A. Proper selection and of test survey instruments.

B. Proper selection of other necessary equipment such as smears, clean taped cork, radiation tags and ribbon, marking pencil, smear sheet, etc.

C. Proper use of floor plan or smear sheet for survey planning and record keeping.

D. Proper survey technique with instruments used. (Use of headphones emphasized.)

E. Smear counting and record keeping. (Knows fraction to be alpha counted. Trainee is aware of places where alpha emitters are expected.)

F. Isolation and proper tagging of contamination, buildings, areas, or equipment.

G. Notification of area supervisor if above is necessary.

H. Proper HP log entry concerning survey results and action taken.

V. Decontamination Procedure

A. Knows recommended procedure for decontaminating personnel and personal clothing.

B. Knows recommended procedure for decontaminating floors, building, and equipment.

VI. Safe Work Permit Coverage

Has participated with a senior health physicist in at least ten jobs requiring Safe Work Permits. Specific attention will be given to:

A. Obtaining adequate information about the job and about how much the workmen know about it.

B. Direct radiation hazards:

1. Locating hot spots in work areas.

2. Obtaining information concerning the dose status of each workman.

3. Determining radiation type, measuring dose-rate and estimating "working field." (Including hand dosages).

4. Calculating work time on basis of estimate. (This includes hand doses)

5. Making sure that he and all workmen are wearing film badges and dosimeters properly, with instructions to workmen for use.

6. If monitoring is to be intermittent, specifies to workmen when the HP should be recalled to the job.

7. When monitoring is continuous, the HP calls out changes in the radiation field and calls a halt to work when necessary.

     ___ ___ ___ ___ ___ ___

C. Contamination Hazards

1. Locating or anticipating radioactive contamination in the work area.

     ___ ___ ___ ___ ___ ___

2. Advising on the use of blotting paper and/or plastic, etc., to cover work area floors and equipment when necessary and feasible.

     ___ ___ ___ ___ ___ ___

3. Always questions the possibility that the "drained" pipe about to be cut into will contain some radioactive liquid and has plans made to catch it.

     ___ ___ ___ ___ ___ ___

4. Checks frequently to ascertain that contamination is being confined to the area intended.

     ___ ___ ___ ___ ___ ___

5. Monitors for air contamination:

a. Can position and operate a HV Air Sampler and calculate c/cc of air monitored, and find RCG for isotopes found at plant.

     ___ ___ ___ ___ ___ ___

b. Has demonstrated his ability to analyze CAM charts and calculate T 1/2 and aau.

     ___ ___ ___ ___ ___ ___

6. Pays attention to proper handling of potentially contaminated tools and equipment which must be removed from the work area.

     ___ ___ ___ ___ ___ ___

7. Observes habits of personnel working on jobs with possible radioactive contamination, recommends procedures for contamination control, and makes thorough contamination survey of individual when he leaves such a job.

     ___ ___ ___ ___ ___ ___

8. Knows radioactive clothing confiscation procedure.

     ___ ___ ___ ___ ___ ___

D. Has demonstrated proficiency in the proper use of and handling procedure for Anti-C clothing and respiratory equipment with special attention to the following:

1. Replacement (not covering) of personal clothing with Anti-C coveralls.

     ___ ___ ___ ___ ___ ___

2. Selection and use of gloves.

     ___ ___ ___ ___ ___ ___

3. Selection and use of shoe covers.

     ___ ___ ___ ___ ___ ___

4. Proper removal of Anti-C clothing and respiratory equipment to prevent the spread of contamination.

     ___ ___ ___ ___ ___ ___

5. Can quickly assemble, put on and properly fit and leak test the following respiratory protective devices:

	Satisfactory Performance Reviewer's Initials					
	MTR	ETR	ATR	CPP	CFA	TAN

    a. Comfo (or other) half-face filter respirator.

    b. Assault Mask (or other) full face filter respirator.

    c. Scott Air Pak

    d. Airline Respirator

  6. Is familiar with the storage locations of area respiratory equipment.

  7. Knows proper use of above respiratory equipment, including limitations, peculiarities, etc.

E. Completes HP part of Safe Work Permit, distributes information properly and discusses recommendations with workmen.

F. Makes proper log entries concerning the job.

G. Knows when and how to complete plant incident reports.

At this point the technician qualifies to monitor for and sign Safe Work Permits   (Date)

VII. Shipping Procedure

A. Has done the necessary HP work on at least 6 outgoing "on site" readioactive shipments and 10 outgoing "off site" radioactive shipments.

B. Has done the necessary HP work on at least 6 incoming "on site" radioactive shipments and 10 incoming "off site" radioactive shipments.

C. Knows proper procedure for shipment of area hot waste dumpster. Specific attention is to ge given to:

    1. Proper completion and distribution of the correct number of hot waste forms.

    2. Correct calculation of hot waste dumpster curie content.

    3. Checking the radiation dose rate in the dumpster truck cab.

At this point the technician has met the requirements necessary for authorization to ship and receive radioactive materials   (Date)

VIII. Instrumentation

A. Knows location of all fixed health physics monitoring instruments.

B. Knows proper procedure for inspecting the above instruments and initialing the charts.

	MTR	ETR	ATR	CPP	CFA	TAN
C. Knows proper procedure for tagging out inoperative instruments and submitting instrument repair work orders.	___	___	___	___	___	___
D. Can perform secondary calibration (sensitivity) check on the following:						
1. Constant Air Monitors (CAMs)	___	___	___	___	___	___
2. Radiation Area Monitors (RAMs)	___	___	___	___	___	___
3. Portal Monitors	___	___	___	___	___	___
4. Beta-Gamma Hand & Foot Counter	___	___	___	___	___	___
5. Alpha Hand & Foot Counter	___	XXX	XXX	XXX	___	XXX
6. Stack Gas Monitor	___	___	___	___	XXX	___
7. Effluent Water Monitors or samplers	___	XXX	XXX	___	___	___
8. Stack Particulate Monitor	___	___	___	___	___	___
9. Calciner Solid Storage CAM	___	___	___	___	___	___
10. Calciner Ruthenium Absorber and Calculation of Ruthenium Activity	XXX	XXX	XXX	___	XXX	XXX
11. CF Laundry Clothing Monitoring Table	XXX	XXX	XXX	XXX	___	XXX
E. Can perform primary calibration checks on the following:						
1. Constant Air Monitors (CAMs)	___	___	___	___	___	___
2. Radiation Area Monitors (RAMs)	___	___	___	___	___	___
3. Alpha Hand & Foot Counters	___	XXX	XXX	___	___	___
4. Stack Gas Monitor	___	___	___	___	___	___
5. Stack Particulate Monitor	___	___	___	___	___	___
6. Hood Exhause Monitor	___	XXX	XXX	___	___	___
7. Iodine Fission Break Monitor	___	___	___	___	XXX	XXX
8. Calciner Solid Storage CAM	XXX	XXX	XXX	___	XXX	XXX
9. Calciner Ruthenium Absorber and Calculation of Ruthenium Activity	XXX	XXX	XXX	___	XXX	XXX
F. Knows limits and procedures for reporting Stack Monitor Effluent Discharge.	___	___	___	___	___	___
G. Can operate a gamma scintillation spectrometer and:						
1. Identify the isotopes which commonly appear at the plant where he works.	___	___	___	___	___	___
2. Can determine the amount of activity in a sample by photopeak analysis for the same isotopes.	___	___	___	___	___	___
H. Can operate thyroid counter and determine the approximate dose.	___	___	___	___	___	___

1388

	MTR	ETR	ATR	CPP	CFA	TAN

IX. Water Samples

    A. Where applicable collects routine water samples, and fills out forms correctly.

    B. Where applicable prepares daily routine water samples, uses pipette correctly, counts samples, calculates half-life, and keeps proper records of same.

X. Source Storage

    A. Knows locations of radioactive sources in the area.

    B. Knows proper procedure for locating, inventory, and leak checking the radioactive sources in the area.

XI. Ventilation

    A. Has a working knowledge of the area ventilation system.

    B. Can determine hood velocities and knows proper tag-out procedure for those not meeting specifications.

XII. Emergency Action Plan

    A. Has read, is familiar with, and knows location of the Emergency Action plans for the area.

    B. Knows signals for evacuation and alert.

    C. Knows location of area evacuation signal and how to operate it.

    D. Knows where area emergency equipment cabinets, change areas, showers, etc., are located.

XIII. NRTS Burial Grounds

    A. Knows procedures for burying materials, record-keeping, and preparation of Burail Ground plot plan.

	MTR	ETR	ATR	CPP	CFA	TAN
A.	XXX	XXX	XXX			XXX

    B. Knows proper procedure for handling burial of classified shipments.

	MTR	ETR	ATR	CPP	CFA	TAN
B.	XXX	XXX	XXX	XXX		XXX

XIV. Is familiar with HP problems and procedures of CF Radioactive Laundry operation.

XV. X-Ray Diffraction Units

    A. Is familiar with the fundamentals of X-Ray Diffraction Unit operations.

	MTR	ETR	ATR	CPP	CFA	TAN
A.					XXX	

    B. Is familiar with the hazards associated with X-Ray Diffraction Units.

	MTR	ETR	ATR	CPP	CFA	TAN
B.					XXX	

	Satisfactory Performance Reviewer's Initials					
	MTR	ETR	ATR	CPP	CFA	TAN

XVI. Radiographic X-Ray Machines

    A. Is familiar with Radiographic Standard
       Practices on X-ray machines. ___ ___ ___ ___ ___ ___

    B. Is familiar with the hazards associated with
       radiographic X-ray machines. ___ ___ ___ ___ ___ ___

    C. Is familiar with the hazards and techniques
       associated with the use of radiography sources. ___ ___ ___ ___ ___ ___

XVII. Has received the proper training and has shown
the necessary proficiency for the responsibilities
of an HP technician in all phases of nonradiological
safety as prescribed by the H & S Safety Section
(TO BE INITIALED BY SAFETY ENGINEER). ___ ___ ___ ___ ___ ___

XVIII. Other on-the-job advanced training or duties satisfactorily performed (list area)

_____

_____

_____

XIX. Additional formal education under NRTS or other programs.

Course No.   School   Course Title   Completed

_____

_____

INC HEALTH PHYSICS TRAINING CHECK LIST   Exhibit (C)
PROGRESS REPORT

Date _____   Area _____

I.	Orientation
	Items A - 1 & 2
	Item A - 3 (HP Class)
	Item A - 4 (1st Aid Course)
	Item A - 5
	Item B
	Item C
II.	Green Tag Authorization
III.	Radiation Surveys
IV.	Contamination Surveys
V.	Decontamination Procedure
VI.	Safe Work Permit HP Coverage
VII.	Shipping Procedure
	Items A - B
	Item C
VIII.	Instrumentation
	Items A - C
	Item D
	Item E
	Item F
	Item G
	Item H
IX.	Water Samples
X.	Source Storage
XI.	Ventilation
XII.	Emergency Action Plan
XIII.	NRTS Burial Grounds
XIV.	HP Aspects - CF Laundry
XV.	X-Ray Diffraction Units
XVI.	Radiographic X-Ray Machines
XVII.	Nonradiological Safety
XVIII.	Other on the Job Training
XIX.	Additional Formal Education
XX.	Other Plants Qualified In:
	ATR
	ETR
	MTR
	TAN
	CFA
	CPP

Periodically health physics technicians are shifted from one plant to another. Such a change of assignment requires him to train for that particular plant in accordance with the check list, but does not officially reduce the technician to trainee.

Since it is very important that plant HP technicians be thoroughly familiar with their assigned plant, the IN technician training check list includes this point. To aid the technicians in this familiarization requirement, an internal training manual was compiled for this purpose. This manual gives a general description of the specific plants and areas emphasizing radiation hazards and safety procedures.

ISU RADIATION PROTECTION TECHNOLOGY COURSE

Because of the increasing industrial demand for trained health physics technician level personnel, the AEC-IDAHO Operations Office (ID), Idaho State University and the Idaho Nuclear Corporation began a joint venture in 1965 to train such technicians. (Idaho Nuclear replaced Phillips Petroleum Company at the NRTS in this capacity on July 1, 1966.) With the agreement that a basic science two-year college man made a good technician, ISU developed a "Radiation Protection Technology" (RPT) two-year curriculum. The program includes two years of academic training at ISU and two summers of training under IN Health Physics at the NRTS. The two year ISU curriculum is fully accredited and allows a student to apply his credits to a BS degree if he wishes.

The summer training was initially an expansion of the program used for IN technician training. It is now a much broader based program which attempts to train HP technicians for any work demanding radiation safety control services. It is anticipated that these technicians will frequently have no technical health physics or safety personnel to turn to during emergency situations. Therefore, their understanding of university health physics, medical health physics, licensee laboratory, and industrial safety problems must be more extensive.

Since the ISU-RPT technicians may eventually work in other areas and programs besides those controlled by IN, an attempt is made to give the student a broader fund of knowledge and training. The academic training at ISU is as follows:

First Year: Biology, Mechanical Drawing, AEC Orientation, Introduction to Chemistry, English Composition, Algebra, Trigonometry, Calculus, Analytical Geometry, Speech, Electives.

Second Year: Introduction to Probability, Physics, Physical Education, Human Relations, Materials and Processes, English Composition, Expository Writing, Electives.

ISU-RPT TRAINEE
SUMMER CLASSROOM TRAINING

The first 13 week summer of the ISU-RPT program at the NRTS is mostly classroom training designed to familiarize the students with the basic principles of radiation protection and introduce them

HEALTH PHYSICS TECHNICIAN TRAINING 1393

ISU Radiation Protection Technology Program
Summer Training Course (2nd Year)

June 10 - September 6, 1968

7th Week - Starting July 22	
In-Plant Training(TAN-CPP)- M. L. Arave 29hrs	In-Plant Training(MTR-ETR)-D. Majors 23 hrs
Special Assignments - 11 hrs	Special Assignments - 17 hrs
Monday, July 22 3:30 - 4:30 P.M. - Seminar #4 (MTR 667)	Monday, July 22 3:30 - 4:30 P.M. - Seminar #4 (MTR 667)
Tuesday, July 23 12:30 - 1:30 P.M. - Toxicology - (MTR 667) (P. B. Anderson) ·1:30 - 2:30 P.M. - Ventilation and Radiation Safety - (MTR 667) - D. D. Coward 2:30 - 4:30 P.M. - Methods in First Aid - L. L. Berry -	Tuesday, July 23 12:30 - 1:30 P. M. - Toxicology - (MTR 667) (P. B. Anderson) 1:30 - 2:30 P.M. - Ventilation and Radiation Safety - (MTR 667) - D. D. Coward 2:30 - 4:30 P.M. - Methods in First Aid - L. L. Berry -
Thursday, July 25 12:30 - 2:30 P.M. - Ventilation and Radia- tion Safety - D. D. Coward - 2:30 - 4:30 P.M. - Methods in First Aid - L. L. Berry -	Thursday, July 25 12:30 - 2:30 P.M. - Ventilation and Radiation - D. D. Coward 2:30 - 4:30 P.M. - Methods in First Aid - L. L. Berry -
Any time during the week . . . . Review of Protective Breathing Equipment - 2 hours -	Any time during the week . . . . 1. Review of Protective Breathing Equip- ment ------------------------------ 2hrs 2. Radon-Thoron Activity Problem ------ 6hrs
Group I - (MTR-ETR)	Group II - (CPP-TAN-CFA)
8th Week - Starting July 29	
In-Plant Training - D. Majors - 23-1/2 hrs	In-Plant Training - M. L. Arave - 26-1/2 hrs
Special Assignments - 16-1/2 hrs	Special Assignments - 13-1/2 hrs
Tuesday, July 30 12:30 - 2:30 P.M. - Expectations of HP in Fire Fighting - MTR 667 - AEC Fire Dept. 2:30 - 4.30 P.M. - Methods in First Aid - L. L. Berry -	Tuesday, July 30 12:30 - 2:30 P.M. - Expectations of HP in Fire Fighting - MTR 667 - AEC Fire Dept. 2:30 - 4:30 P.M. - Methods in First Aid - L. L. Berry -
Thursday, August 1 9:30 - 12 A.M. - Fire Fighting and Radia- tion Safety Problem - AEC Fire Dept. 12:30 - 2:30 P.M. - Ventilation and Radia- tion Safety 2:30 - 4:30 P.M. - Methods in First Aid - L. L. Berry -	Thursday, August 1 9:30 - ·12 A.M. - Fire Fighting and Radia- tion Safety Problem - AEC Fire Dept. 12:30 - 2:30 P.M. - Ventilation and Radia- tion Safety 2:30 - 4:30 P.M. - Methods in First Aid - L. L. Berry -
Any time during the week . . . . MTR Chapter Questions and Answers ------- 3 hours Spectrometer Familiarization ------- 3 hours - J. L. Clark -	Any time during the week . . . . CPP Chapter Questions and Answers -------- 3 hours

to the training areas used for the second summer program. They are also given an opportunity to get a
good understanding of HP technician work at this time.
The classroom training is more extensive than the
session given IN trainees. The teaching staff is
primarily the same as that of the IN program with
university guest lecturers and AEC training personnel
and facilities being used to help broaden the course.

ISU-RPT IN-PLANT TRAINING

The purpose of the second 13 week summer
training period for the ISU-RPT students at the NRTS
is to provide intensive in-plant training. The class is
divided into training groups of three to five students.
Each group is assigned to an IN controlled area for a
scheduled period of training time depending on the
number of training groups. The schedule allows all
groups to train an equal amount of time in each area.
Each group is assigned to an experienced HP specialist in each area who devotes full time to in-plant
training using a check list similar to the IN check list
but modified to better serve the needs of the ISU
program. The specialist shifts the group from assignment to assignment as conditions warrant, insuring
that they get involved in as many health physics and
safety projects as is practical.
Supplementary training exercises are projected
on paper using the plant area as a background. These
problems are discussed, solved and critiqued by each
group. This gives them an opportunity to become acquainted with some conditions that might not arise
during their stay in the area. Also interspersed with

the in-plant training are seminars required of each trainee, advanced instruction in instrument usage, specific instruction on non-radiological industrial hygiene problems, staged fire fighting problems involving radiation sources and several other demonstrative training sessions. A portion of a typical training schedule is reproduced as a Exhibit D.

Each point in the trainee's check list must be initialed by the training HP specialist before credit can be given for training completion.

At the end of the second summer training period, each student is given an oral examination and evaluated by a panel of competent health physics supervisors, foremen, and senior technicians. The results from these exams indicate that a high degree of competence has been achieved by the students in the program.

ISU TECHNICIAN CERTIFICATION

Upon satisfactory completion of two years, i. e., 64 semester hours of approved selected material at ISU, IN classroom and in-plant training at NRTS, the trainees are granted a joint certificate by Idaho State University, the Atomic Energy Commission and Idaho Nuclear Corporation.

NRTS HEALTH PHYSICS
PROFICIENCY CERTIFICATION

December 18, 1968, the final stamp of approval was placed on a health physics technician certification program by the University of Idaho through the University of Idaho NRTS Education Program.

This program is open to all AEC contractors at the NRTS. Requirements for certification are as follows:

Academic Requirements

Subject	Minimum Semester Hours Credit
Biological Science	3
Engineering Graphics	2
Chemistry	3
English Composition	3
College Algebra	3
Speech	2
Technical Writing	3
Intro Management Theory	3
Physics	3
Radiological Health	6
	31

Training Requirements

An acceptable classroom or equivalent training period, completion of an in-plant training check list and passage of an oral examination are also required. Upon completion of this program the sponsoring institution issues a health physics proficiency certificate.

Note: The program is indebted to the Public Health Program for its early work in Radiation Safety Control training programs and its training publications, particulary the Radiological Health Handbook.

REFERENCES

1. H. W. Stroschein, and P. H. Maeser, eds.,
   Health Physics Technician Training Manual, IDO-
   17182, Phillips Petroleum Company, Atomic Energy Division, National Reactor Testing Station, U.S.
   Atomic Energy Commission, June 1966.

2. OP cit p iii

HEALTH PHYSICS INDOCTRINATION
AND RE-INDOCTRINATION OF
IDAHO NUCLEAR CORPORATION EMPLOYEES*

P. H. Maeser, E. A. King,
H. W. Stroschein, and J. W. McCaslin
Idaho Nuclear Corporation
Idaho Falls, Idaho

ABSTRACT

All new employees of Idaho Nuclear Corporation
are required to attend a health physics indoctrination
lecture. The presentation is devised to satisfy legal
requirements, allay fears, correct misconceptions,
acquaint employees with basic concepts of radiation
and radiation protection, and familiarize them with
company policies and plant procedures. The lecture
includes the basic concepts of radiation, units of radiation measurement, biological effects of radiation,
principles of radiation protection, contamination control procedures with demonstrations showing proper
methods of donning and removing anticontamination
clothing, and procedures to follow during emergencies.

---

*Work performed under the auspices of the Atom-
ic Energy Commission.

The Health Physics re-indoctrination program
provides an annual review of some aspects of radiation safety procedures and policies for all Idaho Nuclear Corporation personnel working in radiation
areas, and acquaints them with recent changes in radiation protection procedures. The re-indoctrination
also provides a chance to ask questions on radiation
safety that the employees did not have the opportunity,
knowledge or experience to ask on previous occasions.
The presentation is varied from year to year as specific needs become apparent. These orientation lectures have increased job efficiency, decreased contamination spread, lowered radiation exposure and
resulted in better rapport between the average employee and the health physics department.

INTRODUCTION

Idaho Nuclear Corporation (IN) is a subsidiary
corporation of Aerojet General and Allied Chemical
Corporations operating under an Atomic Energy Commission (AEC) contract at the National Reactor Testing Station (NRTS) located near Idaho Falls, Idaho.
The contracted operation includes three large test
and experimental reactors, a chemical processing
plant, a radioactive waste calciner, two large decontamination facilities, several hot cells, and caves,
numerous chemical laboratories, and the general
services for all site contractors. The employees number 2,000 with approximately 220 full time and part
time new employees being hired annually.
The primary goal of a good safety program is to
prevent accidents. Idaho Nuclear Corporation

conducts two indoctrination programs in radiation
safety to help accomplish this goal, i. e. , the indoctrination of all new employees in basic radiation safety
procedures and an annual health physics re-indoctrination for all employees.

HEALTH PHYSICS INDOCTRINATION
FOR NEW EMPLOYEES

The indoctrination presentation is designed to
serve serveral purposes:

1. It covers specific topics and insures a uniform
   introduction to radiation problems and written
   procedures for all new employees.

2. It satisfies legal requirements.

3. It allays fears and misconceptions in reference to radiation.

4. The new employee is introduced to company
   policies and plant procedures so that he can
   work with a minimum of worry and inefficiency.

5. Background knowledge of the basic concepts
   of radiation and radiation protection is provided the employee so that he can meet new
   or unexpected events intelligently.

6. The presentation must change from group to
   group depending upon the level of understanding of the least informed.

7. The new employees are given some idea of
   how to proceed in case an emergency involves
   their work area.

8. New employees are introduced to the health physics group as a service organization and informed that this group should be contacted for radiation safety advice.

The indoctrination procedure starts with a 15 to 20 minute "Pre-indoctrination" on the first day of employment. This is followed by a more complete presentation three to five days later, which lasts two and one half hours. The "pre-indoctrination" introduces the new employees to the basic procedures of personnel dosimetry, radiation ribbons, alarming radiation instruments, and evacuation sirens to the extent that they can work around radiation, if necessary, with a minimum of instructions.

The contents of the indoctrination lecture are divided into six sub-divisions. The first pertains to the basic concepts of radiation. Employees learn that radiation is a universal phenomenon co-existent in time with the universe, omnipresent on the earth's surface and not to be feared per se. This is accomplished by briefly defining and reviewing the different types of radiation and comparing them with ionizing radiation and showing similarities in the methods of protection from each. Introduction is made to the basic kinds of ionizing radiation and their characteristics from a health physics standpoint. The inability of our five senses to warn us of the presence of ionizing radiation is stressed at this stage with the fact that we must have instrumentation to detect the hazard for us. The alleviation of any fears of new employees is considered to be quite important. Any indication of fear is given special consideration at this time and discussed accordingly. This may require extra time

with the individual after the lecture; however, it is
usually taken care of by special consideration during
the remainder of the presentation.

The second area of discussion is on the basic units
and methods of measuring ionizing radiation. The
roentgen and the roentgen equivalent man measurement units are explained to the degree necessary to
clarify them for all in attendance. At this point, a
demonstration is conducted on how radiation is detected and measured with instrumentation. Alpha,
beta, and gamma sources of low magnitude are measured with a portable alpha meter and a low range
"GM" meter connected to an audio amplifier, as the
detectors and the source characteristics are demonstrated and discussed. The comparative amounts and
kinds of material needed to shield alpha, beta, and
gamma are also demonstrated at this time.   The
sources used (a chip of plutonium-aluminum alloy,
a one ml glass dish with evaporated ^{90}Sr contaminated water, and a 1/4" ^{60}Co wire) help make the
employee aware of the fact that the least suspected
items may be radioactive and that an instrument is
necessary to detect it. Shielding materials as well as
time in the field and distance from the source factors
are demonstrated at this time to convince the new employee that one can protect himself and work around
radiation safely. Radiation dose and dose-rate are also
covered at this time.

Reference is made to the biological effects of
radiation as the third item in the indoctrination. It is
not covered in great detail, but enough is mentioned
to enable the employee to understand the hazards involved in working carelessly around radiation. Some
of the expected effects of certain acute whole-body

radiation doses for humans are mentioned to give the
employee an idea of the acute dose required to bring
about harmful effects. These acute exposure effects
vs the effects of an accumulated dose from exposures
over a longer period of time are included in this discussion. The administrative RPG's are listed and the
safety factor emphasized to show the employee that
he need not worry about any biological effects if he
works properly.

At this stage of the orientation the new employees
are ready to consider the procedures and policies for
radiation safety. The principles of radiation protection
are covered with specific references and examples
showing how time, distance, and shielding are used
while working with radiation. If the lecturer has done
a good job in covering the subject as outlined to this
point, he has very little trouble in getting those in attendance to accept the specific procedures as he lists
them. The fact that special plant procedures will be
necessary depending upon the plant operation and the
practices of the HP supervisor is stressed and the
plant HP's are recommended as the best sources for
learning of these procedures.

The protection from contamination is discussed by
showing specific examples of anti-contamination clothing and demonstrating its proper use on a manikin. A
mock contaminated area is used to exhibit the proper
use of radiation warning tags and ribbons and the recommended procedure for removing shoe covers when
leaving such an area is demonstrated. The removing
of possibly contaminated latex gloves by turning them
inside out is also shown. The procedures for the
proper use of respiratory system protective equipment is explained and the importance of the face

piece being properly fitted to the face is emphasized.
Area and personnel decontamination procedures are
treated with special reference to the possibilities of
harmful effects if contamination is not cleaned up.
References to procedures in disposal of radioactive
waste are also made.

Evacuation procedures and policies are covered
as the sixth subdivision of the indoctrination. A sample evacuation route sign is shown and the details explained for each IN contracted area. All employees
are expected to know that the procedure does vary
from plant to plant and since any employee may be
assigned to work in any plant area the individual responsibility for plant evacuation knowledge is stressed.
The "Idaho Nuclear Emergency Action Plan" book is
referenced for their source of this information.

The lecture is presented with the aid of a set of
14" x 22" flash cards and a 8 1/2" x 11" page size
three ring binder containing pictures of such things as
hand and foot counters, portal monitors, and samples
of radiation warning tags. The presentation must be
made by an individual who enjoys teaching to make it
successful. This individual must know the subject
sufficiently well to present it on a proper level for
those in attendance and must not become bored by the
monotony of repetition. The attitude toward the presentation by the lecturer is that personnel are being
informed on something worthwhile, their health. The
assignment of just any health physics employee to
present this lecture results in a waste of time for both
the lecturer and those in attendance.

The lecture concludes with a question and answer
period and the distribution to all personnel in attendance of a booklet, "Play It Cool With Radiation,"

which reiterates the lectural discussion and serves
as a reference pamphlet.

Plans for the future of the indoctrination lecture
include the addition of a large training board containing such signals as the evacuation siren, constant
air monitor alarms, the alert siren, fire alarm, and
portal monitor alarms. This will enable the instructor
to introduce the new employee to the sounds of these
important warning devices, and not just talk about
them.

ANNUAL HEALTH PHYSICS
RE-INDOCTRINATION PROGRAM

In addition to the indoctrination lecture for all
new employees, an annual health physics re-indoctrination lecture is given to other IN employees.
The primary purpose of this program is to help prevent radiation accidents by requiring employees to
focus their minds on radiation safety for approximately thirty to forty minutes each year. The presentation reviews some phase or phases of the initial
indoctrination in more depth, therefore, refreshing
the employee's memory in the keeping of certain procedures and principles for safety sake. Other purposes
are served as well. Changes in health physics administrative practices and procedures can be introduced
and stressed in such a way that the major portion of
the employees will hear about it from a well-informed
source, not by rumor or hear-say. For example, in
1968, a new evacuation procedure for one of the IN
contracted areas was introduced and discussed in ad-

dition to the material prepared for review. The presentation period also provides an opportunity for dia-
logue between other workers and the health physics
group. They can question, cajole, gripe, argue about
any specific procedure that puzzles them. This has
resulted in some changes of procedure and improvement of personnel moral.

The presentation is given each year during the
months of October, November, and December. Several
presentations are scheduled in each contracted area
for the convenience of shift workers. All employees
working in hazardous or potentially hazardous radiation areas any amount of time during the year are
expected to attend one of the annual re-indoctrination
sessions. It is estimated that about 75% of the employees attend each year. An occasional absence is
tolerated, but habitual absentees are given a wrist-
slap or a reminder by their supervisors. An attendance roster is circulated for all to sign and a permanent attendance record kept on the individual employee
exposure cards.

In order to be effective each year, it is necessary
that the topics vary and that repetition be held to a
minimum. During the past few years topics covered
have been such items as internal radiation exposure
control, basis for administrative exposure limits,
recommended anti-C clothing procedure, and basic
radiation safety information.

The methods of presentation also vary from year
to year. Lectures with visual aids, recently released
health physics movies, demonstrations, and questionnaires are perhaps the most popular methods of
presentation in our program. A radioactive contami-

nation control demonstration received numerous
favorable comments a few years ago. The demonstration showed how fast and easy it is to spread contamination. A small area of the lecture room containing a small table, a couple of chairs, writing
tablets, and pencils was ribboned off with magenta
and yellow ribbon and clearly labeled with radiation
warning tags. The floor area, furniture, and writing
materials were contaminated with silver activated
zinc sulfide. The attendance group was kept to a maximum number of forty with five of them volunteering
to help with the demonstration. They were asked to go
into the ribboned area for various reasons which involved the need for pencil and paper. Anti-C clothing
was provided for proper dressing under the labeled
conditions of the area. Upon their return from the
area, in most cases with a sheet of the provided paper,
they were checked for contamination with an ultra
violet light. Then the volunteer performers were
asked to remove their anti-C clothing. As they removed the clothing, intermittent contamination spread
checks were made. This did a good job in demonstrating that regardless of how careful an individual is in
removing the clothing, it can still spread to the skin
and personal clothing and therefore, it is always a
good idea to get checked out by a radiation detector
instrument. In one case, it demonstrated that it
doesn't pay to borrow a chair from a contaminated
marked area. The thief was identified with the aid of
the ultra violet light and the beautiful florescence in
the sit-down region of his trousers. This demonstration must be dramatically explained by the lecturer as
it progresses for maximum effect. Zinc sulfide demonstrations of other sorts have been as effective.

Other examples of successful presentations in the program include the film "Radiation in Perspective" the year it was released for showing, emphasizing the fact that it was available for public showing, a radiation knowledge questionnaire, and a lecturer utilizing transparencies and an overhead projector.

The annual re-indoctrination has done a variety of things since its inception. It is felt that it has increased rapport between Health Physics and the other working groups, decreased contamination spread, decreased unnecessary radiation exposure, increased employee knowledge about health physics procedures and radiation principles, increased health physics awareness of other groups' problems, and served as a snoozing period for the maladjusted.

The indoctrination and re-indoctrination presentations have proven to be well worth the time and trouble and almost mandatory for any operation where radiation is handled.

SHORT COURSES IN EMERGENCY MONITORING FOR SAFETY AND MEDICAL PERSONNEL

R. R. Landolt and P. L. Ziemer
Bionucleonics Department, Purdue University
Lafayette, Indiana

INTRODUCTION

Training courses in radiation safety for personnel whose work is either directly or indirectly involved with ionizing radiation are not unusual. In
fact many, perhaps most, health physicists find that
one of their more important functions is to provide
radiation safety training on an informal or a formal
basis to a variety of individuals. Our purpose in discussing short courses for safety and medical personnel is not with the idea that the presenting of such
courses is a novel idea, nor that the course content
that we used is somehow unique. Rather we wish to
emphasize the responsibility of the practicing health
physicist to use short courses or similar training
techniques as a means of integrating other health and
safety personnel in his facility into the radiation
safety program, particularly with respect to planning
for radiation emergenices. Perhaps this is a more
pronounced need at our institution in that our health

physics group is not administratively a part of either
the University Safety and Security Department or of
the University Health Service. Such is not always the
case; indeed, at many institutions and facilities, the
health physics group is directly a part of another
safety and/or medical organization. Nevertheless,
the general principles of utilizing such training will
apply in most situations, although we will necessarily
evaluate such training from our own perspective.

TEAM PLANNING FOR EMERGENCIES

It has been pointed out in the past (1) that in emergency planning, the health physics team must work
closely with safety, fire, and medical personnel in
an installation in order to coordinate radiation emergency activities and to acquaint all concerned with the
types of hazards and potential emergencies peculiar
to the installation in question. Safety personnel, especially the fire department, need to be provided with
not only the general fundamental knowledge about radiation hazards, but also with specific information on
the locations of radiation and radioisotope areas, and
the types of special precautions required. Likewise
medical personnel need a general understanding of
radiation hazards, and special training on handling
emergencies involving injured persons who are contaminated, individuals who have ingested significant
amounts of activity, or overexposed persons.

Fo coordinate activities in emergency preplanning
and émergency training, we have found it useful to
establish a "Radiation Emergency Committee" which

functions as a subcommittee of our Radiological Control Committee. The emergency committee is composed of representatives from the safety and security staff, the medical staff, and the health physics staff. We have also added a representative from our news bureau, since experience indicates that press releases and public relations are extremely important in radiation accidents or incidents. Such a committee can not only set policies governing emergency situations but can also serve to stimulate and coordinate training programs on emergency monitoring.

TRAINING FOR SAFETY PERSONNEL

In planning an emergency monitoring course for safety and security personnel, one first has to establish what is to be accomplished. The fact that such individuals should receive some sort of training in radiation emergency monitoring is accepted by most health physicists and by most agencies. For example, the International Atomic Energy Agency says in its technical booklet entitled "Training in Radiological Protection: Curricula and Programming":[2]

> "Fire fighters likely to be called to atomic installations must have some knowledge of radiological protection or they risk exposure to radiation which could prove serious. For similar reasons, police officers need some training in the subject."

Beyond this general statement, the IAEA offered only by the suggestion that the training for policemen and firemen should consist of one to two weeks of informational training and on-site demonstrations.

In a study on radiation safety training programs
made for the Atomic Energy Commission by the
Stanford Research Institute,[3] it is emphasized that in
the case of radiation accidents,

> "...firemen and police often must be prepared to
> take remedial action following an accident in-
> volving possible hazards to the general public.
> It is reasonable to expect that such personnel
> would be the first to arrive at the scene of a ra-
> diation accident.... . It is necessary for at least
> some key personnel of local fire, police, and
> health agencies to have a fundamental knowledge
> of radiation safety in order to contain hazards
> until more specialized personnel reach the scene
> of the accident."

Having determined that training for safety and
security personnel is desirable, the question remains
as to what sort of training is needed. In the Stanford
study,[3] the question of course content and approach
has been considered in some detail for municipal firefighters and police. In large cities, training ranges
from 2 hour to 16 hour courses, while in smaller
towns, courses were somewhat longer, ranging from
15 to 26 hours. The course content ranged from those
which provided minimal training to those offering extensive and rather advanced training for both fire
fighters and officers. In most cases, the courses included general introductory material about radiation
and nuclear fundamentals, followed by special instructions on handling specific types of emergency situations. When the brief, minimal course was used, the
departments relied heavily on the availability of outside experts who would arrive on the scene of any

emergency involving radiation and direct the emergency operations.

In examining the approach used by others, and in evaluating our own situation, it seemed clear that although a solid and extensive grounding in radiation fundamentals was desirable, time limitations and variations in the educational backgrounds of the participants would permit only a limited time to be spent on fundamentals. It is not only desirable, but necessary that a significant effort be directed toward specific aspects of dealing with one's own facility. Hence we believe that the most beneficial approach is to utilize a short-term program with minimum technical detail, which provides a brief introduction to the fundamentals of radiation protection and a strong emphasis on practical problems. (For example, an evaluation of how effective their respiratory devices already on hand would be in fighting fires involving airborne radioactivity.)

There are several training aids and sources of information which are useful in planning courses for security personnel, particularly for firefighters.[4-8] These materials are readily adapted to fit one's own particular needs.

An example of a six hour short-course that we have used for our security personnel (campus police and campus fire department) is outlined in Tables 1 and 2. The technical material is summarized in Table 1 while practical aspects are given in Table 2.

TRAINING FOR MEDICAL PERSONNEL

There does not seem to be good agreement as to what role health physics should play in training medical

Table 1.

Introductory lectures on Technical Aspects of Radiation Safety for

Medical and Safety Personnel (2 hours)

Main Topic	Sub-Topics	Suggested Time
Basic Definitions	What is radioactivity? Radiation? Contamination? Types of Radiation	1/4 hour
Benefits of Radiation	Examples of research, industrial and medical uses of radiation	1/4 hour
Radiation Environment	Background; Natural and Man-Made sources	1/4 hour
Quantities & Units	Curies; Roentgens; Rems	1/4 hour
Types of Hazards	External & Internal Hazards Types of Radiation	1/3 hour
Effects of Radiation	Acute and Chronic Exposures Radiation Syndrome Long-term Effects	1/3 hour
Methods of Protection	External (Time, Distance, Shielding) Internal (Protective Clothing, Respiratory Protection)	1/3 hour

personnel in those radiation safety procedures associated with emergencies. There is the implication in much of the literature on radiation emergencies that there will always be an M. D. available who is well versed in radiation hazards and the handling of radiation accident victims. Or, if such an individual is not on hand, certainly a qualified health physicist will be right on hand to give appropriate advice on handling contaminated or overexposed victims. In reality it is easy to imagine situations in which radiation accident victims could be removed to a hospital (or to the campus or laboratory health center) and emergency treatments initiated without either an M. D. trained in radiological safety or a health physicist being present. For this reason, a more realistic approach would be to train selected members of the medical

Table 2.

Practical Aspects of Radiation Safety for Security Personnel (4 hours)

Main Topic	Sub-Topics	Suggested Time
Federal and State Regulations	Regulations governing use of radiation in our facility. Regulation pertaining to emergency personnel (monitoring, posting, reporting)	1/3 hour
Local (University) Regulations	Lines of Authority Regular Monitoring Programs Posting Facilities	1/3 hour
Film	"Fire Fighting in the Nuclear Age"	1/3 hour
Firefighting Problems Involving Radiation	Types of Restricted Areas Potential External Hazards at Purdue Potential Internal Hazards at Purdue Preventing Spread of Contamination Decontamination and Cleanup	1 hour
Police Problems in Radiation Accidents	Control of Crowds Assisting the Injured Other Emergencies	1/2 hour
Emergency Preplanning	Fire Department Responsibilities Police Department Responsibilities Health Physics Responsibilities	1/4 hour
Discussion	(Open)	1/4 hour
Use of Monitoring Equipment (Field Exercises)	Low & High Level Survey Meters Dosimeters	1 hour

staff, such as those at the admitting station, to be able to carry out simple preliminary surveys.

The late Dr. Robert S. Landauer, Sr., in discussing initial surveys of patients admitted to a hospital after a radiation accident said:[9] "Who is to do the sorting of contaminated and uncontaminated individuals? It must be members of some group which is on duty at all times, every day and night." He goes on to suggest that when possible this sorting should be done by physicians or interns; in smaller hospitals where the supply of physicians is low, other staff members such as nurses could be utilized. Landauer further states that a one-hour lecture demonstration once a month would provide adequate training for this purpose. Similarly, he suggested that a decontamination team composed of a physician, one or two nurses, and several orderlies should be trained for assisting in emergencies.

A similar philosophy has been set forth by Saenger[10] who states that each hospital, regardless of size, should have a well planned disaster program which is reviewed and revised yearly. This program he further states, "must be implemented by frequent training programs for physicians, nurses, technicians, and all ancillary personnel." Saengers plan envisions a hospital team which would include a medical Radiation Safety Officer, technicians trained in radiation accidents, and such other physicians as may be necesary. This team would handle monitoring of patients, personnel, and areas; and carry out decontamination. He suggests training x-ray technicians to serve as monitors and training nurses and operating room orderlies to serve in decontamination teams.

In setting up radiation safety training for the medical personnel at our institution, we followed the ideas of Landauer and Saenger. Although we anticipate that normally our health physics staff will be on hand in any emergency to handle screening of contaminated accident victims or to direct decontamination operations, the possibility of an injured and contaminated victim being taken to our health center before the arrival of health physics emergency personnel exists. It was felt that our medical staff required at least the capability of doing monitoring and simple decontamination.

After discussing possible approaches with the administration of our health center, we established a program consisting of introductory lectures and a two phase practical training program. The introductory lectures and Phase I of the practical training were presented to all regular staff members of the Health Center including physicians, nurses, and laboratory technicians. These lectures were intended to serve as a general orientation so that all the staff, whether directly or indirectly involved in an emergency, would have at least a basic knowledge of what they were dealing with. The second phase, which we have not as yet completed, includes additional training in practical monitoring and decontamination techniques for selected members of the medical staff. An outline of the material used in the Introduction and in Phase I is included in Tables 1, and 3. It should be noted that the introductory material as shown in Table 1 was essentially the same as the introductory lecture used with security personnel. The Introduction and Phase I constituted a four hour course, although the material can be readily condensed or expanded to fit various needs and objectives. The outline for Phase II is also shown in Table 4. In our case this will constitute an additional two-hour training session for the personnel selected to participate.

RETRAINING PERSONNEL

Periodic retraining or refresher courses are an obvious necessity for such programs as described herein. Not only does the constant turnover of personnel make this a necessity, but it is needed due to

Table 3.

Practical Aspects of Radiation Safety for Medical Personnel:

Phase I Emergency Planning (2 hours)

Main Topic	Sub-Topics	Suggested Time
Federal and State Regulations	Regulations governing use of radiation in our facility. Regulations pertaining to emergency personnel	1/3 hour
University Regulations	Lines of Authority Regular Monitoring Programs	1/3 hour
Potential Hazards	Potential External Hazards at Purdue Potential Internal Hazards at Purdue	1/3 hour
Medical Aspects of Radiation Accidents	Types of Accidents General Rules for Medical Personnel Emergency Handling of Contaminated Patients Decontamination Procedures and Contamination Control	1/2 hour
Emergency Preplanning	Responsibilities of Medical Personnel Responsibilities of Health Physics	1/2 hour

the fact that these individuals may go for long periods
of time, perhaps years, without using the knowledge
and techniques learned in a short course. The question
is, with what frequency should refresher courses be
conducted? We have not gained sufficient experience
over an extended length of time to establish an optimum
frequency for refresher or retraining sessions. It is
known that some facilities or agencies attempt annual
refresher courses for such peronnel. It would seem
that one should attempt to strike a happy balance between what is feasible in terms of time and health
physics personnel to devote to such training versus
the probability that such training will actually be utilized or even needed. As G. Hoyt Whipple has aptly
stated[11] relative to emergency planning:

   "An enthusiastic emergency planner can so load
   a facility with caches of emergency instruments,

Table 4.

Practical Aspects of Radiation Safety for Medical Personnel:

Phase II. Emergency Monitoring and Decontamination (2 hours)

Main Topic	Sub-Topics	Suggested Time
Use of Monitoring Equipment	Operation of Survey Instruments Care of Survey Instruments Radiation Surveys in Emergencies	3/4 hour
Screening of Accident Victims	Gross Rapid Screening for Contamination Medical Screening Organizing the Screening Process	1/4 hour
Decontamination of Patients	Decontamination Techniques for Skin & Clothes Decontaminating Agents Acceptable Contamination Limits	1/2 hour

Decontamination of
  Facilities
	Decontamination Techniques for
	  Various Surfaces
	Decontaminating Agents
	Acceptable Contamination Limits
		1/2 hour

ambulances, contaminated operating rooms, mobile shields, and disaster monitors that no time, money or energy are left to carry out the function for which the facility was built."

Just so, one could spend so much time training emergency personnel that there is no time left to get on with the routine health physics programs. (Perhaps this would assure that the emergency personnel would be used!) Thus it is necessary for each facility to evaluate its own situation on frequency of training. In our case, we have not found it feasible to repeat these types of courses on more than a two to three year cycle.

DISCUSSION AND EVALUATION

Facilities that do not have their own security and safety forces or medical facilities must consider

seriously their relationships with local hospitals, fire
departments, and police departments. It would appear prudent in many cases to provide at least brief
training courses of the type described for staff members
of these agencies in the community where such a facility is located.

In a number of communities, fire and police personnel have received radiation monitoring training
through various Civil Defense courses. This provides
them with a good background for handling radiation
emergencies but should be supplemented with specific
detailed instructions about types of potential hazards
associated with your particular facility.

Training courses for firemen often pose scheduling
difficulties due to the manner in which the shifts are
set up. One way to resolve this problem is to conduct
the sessions in the fire station (most have some sort of
lecture area) and teach only the on-duty personnel.
The training session is then repeated a day later to
reach the other shift. This arrangement works quite
well except for those occasions when a bell sounds
and the full class disappears in the middle of a sen-
tence!

A proper evaluation of a short course in emergency monitoring should be made in terms of the
ability of the trainees to apply their training in an accident situation. Our experience in this respect is
minimal since accidents of any significance in facilities such as ours are infrequent. We can only say
that, based on personnel comments made by the participants, they generally felt that they had gained a
grasp and a better perspective of radiation hazards,
and felt that they would be able to deal more intelligently with such hazards should the need arise.

REFERENCES

1. P. L. Ziemer, "Emergency Plans at Universities," in Radiation Accidents and Emergencies in Medicine, Research, and Industry, L. H. Lanzl, J. H. Pingel, and J. H. Rust, eds., Chas. C. Thomas, Publisher, Springfield, (1965) p 261.

2. International Atomic Energy Agency, "Training in Radiological Protection: Curricula and Programming," Technical Report Series No. 31, Vienna (1964), p 6.

3. H. M. Vollmer, L. H. Towle, and B. J. Maynard, "Development of a Radiation Safety Training Program for Industrial and Public Service Personnel," Stanford Research Institute, Menlo Park, Calif. (1960).

4. U. S. Dept. of Health, Education, and Welfare, and U. S. Atomic Energy Commission, "Peacetime Radiation Hazards in the Fire Service, Orientation Unit," OE-84014, Circular No. 641, U. S. Government Printing Office, Washington (1961).

5. U. S. Dept. of Health, Education, and Welfare and U. S. Atomic Energy Commission, "Peacetime Radiation Hazards in the Fire Service, Basic Course Study Guide" OE-84021, U. S. Government Printing Office, Washington (1961).

6. U. S. Atomic Energy Commission, "Living with Radiation, Part I, Fundamentals," U. S. Government Printing Office, Washington (1959).

7. U. S. Atomic Energy Commission, "Living with Radiation, Part II, Fire Service Problems," U. S. Government Printing Office, Washington (1959).

8. F. L. Brannigan, "Radiation Safety Primer, Instructor's Handbook," U. S. Atomic Energy Commission, Safety and Fire Protection Branch, Washington, (1960).

9. R. S. Landauer, Sr., "Hospital Preparedness for Handling Contaminated Persons Requiring Medical Care," in Radiation Accidents and Emergencies in Medicine, Research, and Industry, L. H. Lanzl, J. H. Pingel, and J. H. Rust, eds., Chas. C. Thomas, Publisher, Springfield, (1965) p. 125.

10. E. L. Saenger, "Medical Aspects of Radiation Accidents," U. S. Atomic Energy Commission, Washington (1963) pp. 101-107.

11. G. H. Whipple, "Management, Emergency Organizations, Policy and Plans; Emergency Manuals, Training Drills and Exercises," in Radiation Accidents and Emergencies in Medicine, Research, and Industry, L. H. Lanzl, J. H. Pingel, and J. H. Rust, eds., Chas. C. Thomas, Publisher, Springfield, (1965) p. 225.

ORGANIZATION OF A GRADUATE LEVEL HEALTH PHYSICS SURVEY COURSE*

Sydney W. Porter, Jr.**
Chairman, Professional Educational Committee,
Baltimore-Washington Chapter,
Health Physics Society

Michael S. Terpilak
Training and Manpower Development Program
BRH, ECA, PHS, Rockville, Maryland

ABSTRACT

For the past four years, the Baltimore-Washington Chapter of the Health Physics Society in cooperation with the Training and Manpower Development Program, BRH has conducted a 78-hour graduate level health physics survey course as a refresher and a study guide for applicants preparing for the

---

*This course was partially prepared under the USAEC Contract AT(30-1)-3933:

**Present address: Radiation Management Corporation, 101 North 33rd Street, Philadelphia, Pennsylvania 19104

American Board of Health Physics Certification examination.

The course material and agenda encompasses 26 specific topics which cover the major theoretical, operational and practical aspects of Health Physics. The problems associated with the selection and choice of instructors, teaching techniques and methods, reference materials and texts are presented. Solutions to the administrative problems concerned with low-budget funding and directing of such a course are suggested.

The practical need for this type of education and training, along with suggested guidelines for course organization and presentation are discussed.

I. HISTORY

Four years ago several health physicists in the D. C. area studied and worked problems together to prepare for the ABHP Certification Examination. The notes from this endeavor formed the basis for a course that grew from 15 sessions to the present 27 three-hour sessions.

II. INTRODUCTION

The importance of ABHP certification for the professional health physicist needs no justification. The problem is finding the proper course to help prepare to take the certification examination. Since health physics spans many disciplines, it is extremely difficult if not impossible, to find a two semester graduate

level course that covers all major aspects of health
physics, fundamentals, and introduces current advances in the state of the art. Thus the Chapter decided to develop and organize a course for the individuals in the Baltimore-Washington area. This
survey course constitutes a broad refresher. It does
not pretend to supply the student with all the knowledge
he requires to pass the ABHP examination. It is designed to help the student review the field of health
physics, point up student weaknesses, and to present
current developments in the field.

III. PREREQUISITES FOR STUDENTS

In general, the student should be eligible to take
at least Part I of the ABHP examination.

IV. COURSE AGENDA

The agenda is compiled and updated each year by
the Baltimore-Washington Chapter Professional Education Committee. This Committee consists of at least
two senior (CHP) health physicists, (one with depth in
reactor operating experience, one with depth in medical and/or accelerator health physics), one research
oriented health physicist and one professional teacher
(affiliated with a university) of health physics. Appendix I lists the session, name and description of the
current 1968-1969 course agenda.

V. SELECTION OF INSTRUCTORS AND DIRECTOR

Session instructors are picked by the Professional Education Committee for both their outstanding knowledge, experience in a health physics specialty, and for their ability to communicate with the class. Our experience has shown that outstanding specialists in health physics have been very willing to donate their time and services in order to further the profession of health physics. The Committee attempts to select specialists with teaching experience. The instructor must be able to present his lecture and/or problem session to the level and needs of the class. In order to help accomplish this, the Professional Education Committee retains a Course Director who moderates and directs the level and scope of each session. The Director should have a varied practical health physics background in addition to sufficient graduate level education to enable him to substituted and teach most of the classes should the need arise. He should also be a Board certified health physicist (preferably by written examination) so that he can draw from direct experience in guiding the class in their study program.

VI. ORGANIZATION OF THE INDIVIDUAL SESSIONS

A. The Course Director is selected by the Professional Education Committee in late August. The Course Director assists the Committee in selecting the instructors for each class. Personal contact is made requesting and scheduling speakers prior to the first week in September. In addition followup letters are sent to respective speakers prior to their presentation.

B. Speakers are requested to review the suggested reading and problem assignments and to make any changes at least 3 weeks prior to class presentation.

C. Speakers are also requested to submit several quiz questions that can be completed in 1/4 hour. (Experience has shown that many short quizzes are much more effective than 1 or 2 long exams.) The abilities to work a variety of problems, make logical assumptions to save time, and to budget time in an exam, are all very important tools for taking the ABHP Examination.

D. Registration of applicants for the program is initiated about 10 Sept. and students are selected by the Chapter Professional Education Committee by October 10.

E. A list of required text books, suggested reference books, and the first reading and problem assignment are then sent to each student. Appendix II provides a suggested list of texts.

F. The first class begins during the second week in November. Classes continue until 1 week prior to the ABHP examination in June.

G. Reading and problem assignments are distributed to students at least 2 weeks prior to the class.

H. Time schedule of class:

    1. Review of previous class including assigned homework   1/2 hour

2. Quiz on material from previous class	1/4 hour
(Exact time quiz is given varies from class to class.)	
3. Teaching session	1 hour
4. Coffee break	1/4 hour
5. Teaching session	1 hour

I. Experience in the Baltimore-Washington area indicates that Tuesday evening from 7 to 10 p. m. is the most optimum class time. Three hours is about as long as one can expect to keep the classes attention after an 8-hour work day.

J. A review of the previous class is very important. This provides the student with an opportunity to discuss the previous lecture, to ask questions about any unclear items, and to present the answers to the homework problems to the rest of the class for their comment. If possible, the speaker from the previous class will conduct the review.

VII. COSTS OF THE COURSE FOR TWENTY-FIVE STUDENTS

1. Classroom capacity for 30 students, complete with appropriate visual aids such as slide projector, overhead projector, and blackboard. Since the course is presented on a non-profit basis by a professional group, it should not be too difficult to obtain a classroom free of charge. The Bureau of Radiological Health, Training and Manpower Program has very

graciously supplied this facility to the Baltimore-Washington Health Physics Chapter for the last four years.

2. Reproduction of student reading material. This is mainly supplied by each instructor for his own class. There is still a considerable cost in reproducing material for items such as reading assignments and special reference documents, and material. $200

3. Transportation of out-of-town speakers. Some speakers will be unable to have their agency (company or school) subsidize their transportation expenses. 200

4. Compensation for Course Director. 400

5. Supplies and miscellaneous costs. 50

Total $850

6. Income from 25 students at $30 @ $750.

7. Sponsorship from local Health Physics Chapter is $100.

VIII. SUMMARY

Experience during the past 4 years have shown that the health physics survey course presented in the Baltimore-Washington area has been extremely successful. A total of 11 individuals have taken the ABHP Certification Examination through June 1967, with the following results. Seven have successfully completed the written exam; two have successfully completed the oral exam; and two applications have been unsuccessful.

The results for the year 1968 exam are unavailable at this time, thus preventing a complete tabulation of successful applicants up to this time.

The course is continually reviewed by the Professional Education Committee and also reflects critiques submitted by the students participating in the course. The need for such a course is continually re-emphasized by the large student enrollment each year.

APPENDIX I

Session No.	Description
1. Quantities and Units Dr. Harold O. Wyckoff	Radiation quantities, units, symbols and general nomenclature. Detailed definitions with some background information.
2. Radioactivity and Radioactive Decay Dr. Lewis Battist	Decay, activation, equilibrium and derived quantities.
3. Interaction of Radiation with Matter Mr. James Malaro	α, β, γ and some n absorption and interactions, including both collision and radioactive energy loss.
4. Shielding Mr. Charles W. Garret	General review of processes, broad and narrow beam, relaxation length, properties of shielding materials, many calculations.
5. Radiation Biology I Dr. Robert E. George Dr. Norman C. Telles	Basic mechanisms of damage, relative sensitivity of tissues, acute injury, late effects, effects of penetrating and non-penetrating radiation.
6a. Radiation Biology II Dr. James T. Brennan	Application cellular radiobiology in tumor therapy and radiation protection. Effects of high LET radiation.
6b. Civil Defense Mr. Harold Gaut	Organization, personnel and equipment of Civil Defense in coping with nuclear emergencies. Fallout calculations.
7. Measurement of Radiations (Instrumentation) Mr. Thomas P. Loftus	Principals and operations of free air chambers, cavity chambers, GM tubes $\propto$ proportional counters.
8. Measurement of Radiations (Spectroscopy) Mr. Frazier Bronson Dr. Lewis Battist	Principals and operation of solid state detectors in α, β and γ spectrometry.
9. Luminescence Dosimetry Mr. Thomas L. Johnson	Principals and operation of thermo and radio-photoluminescence dosimeters. Practical applications.
10. Mixed Field (γ + n) Radiation Dosimetry Dr. Joseph Sayeg	Theory and practical application of dosimetry techniques in γ + 1/0n fields.
11. Counting Statistics Mr. Robert Bostrom	Applications of statistics to Health Physics measurements.
12. Personnel Monitoring Mr. Joseph M. Brown, Jr. Mrs. Mardalee B. Dickinson	Theory and practice of film badge personnel dosimetry. Techniques of running a film badge service.
13a. Radiochemistry and Associated Bioassay Techniques Dr. Abraham Goldin	Application of radiochemistry to practical Health Physics monitoring such as environmental.
13b. Preparation for the ABHP Exam Dr. Dade W. Moeller	Qualification of applicants, common pitfalls of examiners, question and answer period.
14. Calculations of Dose from Internally Deposited Radionuclides Dr. Thomas G. Mitchell	β and γ dose calculations for a variety of internal emitters. Critical organ concepts.

APPENDIX I (Cont'd)

15. Reactor Health Physics I
Mr. Patrick Howe
Mr. Sydney W. Porter, Jr.

Licensing and pre-operational surveillance, practical power and research reactor Health Physics considerations.

16a. Reactor Health Physics II
Mr. Michael S. Terpilak

Refueling and major overhaul of large power reactor.

16b. Introduction to Accelerator Health Physics
Mr. Walter E. Gundaker

Basic types of accelerators and overall Health Physics problems.

17. Accelerator Health Physics
Mr. Thomas G. Hobbs

Practical problems of LINACS, long term hazards, ozone problems.

18. Laboratory and Facility Design
Dr. Abraham Schwebel

Basic design criteria for hot labs, decontamination facilities, industrial radiography Health Physics problems.

19. Whole Body Counting
Lt. Earl B. Scrom, MSC USN

Types, uses, designs, operations and limitations.

20. X-ray Health Physics
Mr. Peter J. Valaer

Theory of X-ray generators, NCRP #33 calculations, high energy X-ray facilities.

21. Health Physics at Reprocessing Facilities
Mr. Richard B. Chitwood

Criticality hazards, radioeffluent containment, reconcentration and waste disposal.

22. Air Sampling and Respiratory Protection
Mr. Harry F. Schulte

Respiratory protective device design, testing and utilization. Lung models.

23. Nuclear Accidents and Emergencies I
Mr. Michael S. Terpilak
Dr. James E. Martin

Problems in response to emergencies, case studies, summary of past experience.

24. Nuclear Accidents and Emergencies II
Dr. Neil Wald

Medical and Health Physics aspects of personnel injury cases. Followup of the Pittsburgh accelerator accident.

25. Evaluation of the Environment
Mr. Albert P. Kenneke

Philosophy of RPG and action guides, environmental surveillance.

26. Course Review and General Health Physics
Course Directors and
Mr. Sydney W. Porter, Jr.

Overall review of lectures and homework problems.

27. Radiation Protection Criteria and Standards
Dr. Lauriston S. Taylor
Dr. Forrest Western

Historical development and philosophy of present Radiation Protection Standards and recommendations.

APPENDIX II

Textbooks for the Course Entitled
"Preparation Course for the American Board of
Health Physics Certification Examination"

1. Radiation Dosimetry by Attix, et al., Vol. I
   and II, Academic Press 1966. $40.00

2. The Physics of Radiology by H. E. Johns,
   2nd ed, revised 2nd printing, Charles C.
   Thomas, publisher.   23.00

3. Medical Aspects of Radiation Accidents by
   E. L. Saenger, Superintendent of Documents,
   U.S. Government Printing Office, Washing-
   ton 25, D.C.   1.75

4. National Bureau of Standards Handbook
   Number 63   .40
   Number 69   .35
   Number 75   .35
   Number 76 (NCRP Rpt No. 33)   .25
   Number 80   .50
   Number 84   .20
   Number 85 ·   .70
   Number 93   .30
   Number 97   .50

5. NCRP Report No. 29, Exposure to Radiation
   in an Emergency, available from the Section
   of Nuclear Medicine, Department of Phar-
   macology, The University of Chicago, Chicago
   37, Illinois.   .50

6. ICRP Report of Committee II, 1959, Permissible Dose for Internal Radiation, Pergamon
   Press (1960)   5.50

APPENDIX II (Cont'd)

The student should, if possible, obtain all of the required texts by the first class.

The following texts are recommended. Each student should have a copy of the text or easy access to it.

1. Radioisotope Techniques by Oberman & Clark, McGraw Hill, 1960.   11.00

2. Nuclear Radiation Physics by Lapp & Andrews, 3rd ed, Prentice Hall.   13.00

3. Radiation Hygiene Handbook by Blatz, McGraw Hill, 1959.   29.50

4. Nuclear Radiation Detection by Price, 2nd ed., McGraw Hill.   12.75

5. Assessment of Radioactivity in Man, Vol. I, IAEA, Heidelberg.   8.00

6. The Health Physics Journal, Pergamon Press

7. Principles of Radiation Protection by Morgan & Turner, J. Wiley & Sons.   13.95

Session IX

EMERGENCY PLANNING AND EXPERIENCES

Chairmen

JAMES A. HEACOCK
State Dept. of Industrial Relations
Los Angeles, Calif.

JOHN R. HORAN
U.S. Atomic Energy Commission
Idaho Falls, Idaho

THE ROLE OF RADIATION MONITORING
IN EMERGENCY PREPAREDNESS

John A. McBride and Richard E. Cunningham
Division of Materials Licensing
U. S. Atomic Energy Commission

INTRODUCTION

The AEC operates a regulatory program to protect the public health and safety. Applications submitted to the Commission for licensees to use atomic
energy materials are evaluated to determine that
proposed operations are likely to be conducted safely
and in compliance with regulations. It is recognized,
however, that safety regulations, such as those pro-
mulgated by the AEC, cannot eliminate accidents.
They simply set forth criteria which, if followed,
reduce the probability of accidents and limit their
consequences should they occur.

Recognizing that accidents can happen, persons
licensed by the AEC to use atomic energy materials
are required to prepare plans for actions which would
reduce the hazard to health and safety where the possibility of an emergency exists.   For certain

operations, such as nuclear reactors, fuel reprocessing facilities, fuel fabrication facilities, and industrial radiography, emergency plans are required under AEC regulations contained in 10 CFR 34.32, 50.36, 70.24, and 115.25. Other licensees, such as teletherapy operators and radioisotope processors, are required to provide for coping with emergencies as a condition of their license. For the most part, the regulations simply require a licensee to develop his own plans for coping with emergencies which are credible in his operation. The regulations contain few specific requirements for emergency preparedness and allow wide flexibility in the development of these plans. In some instances, such as the operation of a fuel fabrication facility, there are more specific requirements for instrumentation which will warn of accidents, such as accidental criticality.

In order to determine whether or not the current regulatory program is adequate to assure a reasonable degree of emergency preparedness, the AEC has initiated a study which is intended to evaluate the status of emergency capability for those licensed operations subject to 10 CFR Parts 50, 70, and 115. The purpose of the study is to (1) assess the adequacy of the emergency plans, including provisions for emergency monitoring for these licensed operations; (2) determine whether further regulatory requirements or guidelines are appropriate as a basis for improving emergency plans; and (3) develop information which might be used in the drafting of regulations or guidelines if such action is appropriate. The study includes a survey of emergency preparedness of persons licensed under these regulations. The study is not yet completed, and while no conclusions can be drawn at this time, it is expected that the results will indicate whether there is a need for and the nature of any further action by the AEC in the area of emergency monitoring.

With this as background, the following discussions will describe the role of radiation monitoring in emergency plans for AEC-licensed operations. Monitoring is an important part, but only a part, of emergency planning and will be developed in the context of its function in the overall plan.

EMERGENCY PLANNING

The nature of an emergency plan and emergency monitoring capability will, of course, depend on the concept of an emergency. As it is used in the nuclear industry, the term "emergency" seems to be generic and not one which can be defined with precise limits. A radiation emergency can be considered to be a situation resulting from loss of control over radioactive material, or from imminent loss of control as a result of loss of control over a process involving radioactive material. More broadly, it might be considered as any unplanned situation in which radioactive material affects or threatens to affect the health and safety of the public or employees. The circumstances which initiate the emergency cover a wide range of possibilities, such as operational mistakes, equipment failure, and natural disasters. While the circomstances might be unusual with proper planning and analysis, they need not be unforeseen.

The actual emergency phase of any given of circumstances which affects safety can be considered to

cover that period where prompt action is necessary
to protect life and property. It is preceded by an
occurrence phase which encompasses the events that
initiate the emergency and is followed by a recovery
phase where there is time to plan and organize actions
directly toward the recovery from the emergency.
There is ordinarily no clear demarcation between
emergency and recovery phases.

Emergency plans need to be compatible with the
degree of hazard and radioactive materials involved.
They must be developed to cope with emergencies
which are credible in any given operation. The use
of radioactive materials in AEC-licensed programs
presents a sizable range of possible hazards for which
plans for emergencies need to be prepared in advance.
Production and utilization facilities, such as nuclear
reactors and to a lesser extent fuel reprocessing
plants, are believed to present the greatest potential
for hazard in the event of a serious emergency, since
these types of operations could extend the hazard into
the environment beyond the confines of the plant.
Emergencies in these types of operations have the
potential for involving members of the public as well
as employees of a licensee. By far, most licensed
operations do not involve the large amounts of radioactive materials found in production and utilization
facilities. These are unlikely in an accident situation
to result in major problems of safety beyond the confines of the licensee's plant. Proper planning for
dealing with accidents here is nonetheless important.

Within any given type of operation, there will also
be a variety of accidents which are possible. These
range in seriousness from the type of occurrence
which falls just outside standard operating procedures

up to the most severe accident possible. Plan development should take into account both the range of accidents which can occur and the likelihood of their occurrence. The less serious accidents are usually the ones more likely to occur. Therefore, the more serious accidents should not serve as the sole basis for plan development since this tends to invoke counter measures which are much greater than warranted by the more common type of accident. It can lead to emergency plans being ignored for anything less than the most serious accidents. The plan should offer sufficient flexibility and utility to invoke counter-measures which are appropriate but not excessive for the emergency at hand.

An emergency plan should include a number of specific functions, all of which might be necessary to cope with an emergency, depending on its seriousness. More frequently, however, a specific plan will be drawn to meet the requirements of a specific operation and will include only those functions appropriate to dealing with the potential emergencies foreseen for that operation.

Emergency monitoring is a vital part of any plan, since most of the objectives of any well designed plan cannot be accomplished without the information provided by monitoring to serve as a basis for further decision making. Generally speaking, an emergency capability includes:

An analysis of the types of accidents which are credible, as a basis for developing the plans.

An established plan of action to be put into effect in the event of an emergency. The plan should provide sufficient flexibility with the means to dea

with any of the foreseen situations. It should
also include provisions for emergency monitoring.

An emergency organization, including monitoring
and control center teams which have been trained
in the emergency plan.

Protective action levels which define when various emergency procedures should be placed into
effect.

Provisions for liaison with local civil authorities
during the emergency.

A communications network designed to function
effectively during the emergency.

An established program for obtaining the type of
medical assistance which might be necessary in
credible emergencies.

Emergency equipment stocked in designated locations which are expected to be accessible under
any foreseen conditions. The equipment includes
emergency monitoring instruments, communications equipment, and appropriate protective
equipment.

A planned program of training and periodic retraining of personnel to assure a high level of
proficiency in their roles during an emergency.

A system for release of information which should
be made available to the public about the emergency.

ROLE OF EMERGENCY MONITORING

Within this framework of an organization's emergency capability, the function of emergency monitoring is to provide information about the <u>nature</u> and <u>magnitude</u> of the radiation hazard so that appropriate means can be developed to cope with the specific situation. The information provided by emergency monitoring includes the types and quantities of radionuclides involved in the accident, the extent of human exposure expected, the boundaries of the area affected, and how it is affected. The company management in turn uses this information to invoke plans and procedures for countermeasures. Medical personnel use the information for management of patients who have been exposed or contaminated, and the local civil authorities, frequently with State or Federal assistance, use the information to take appropriate countermeasures to minimize danger to life and property in the environs of the accident.

COMPOSITION AND OPERATION OF AN
EMERGENCY ORGANIZATION

Diagram I is a schematic of emergency situation management. It describes the composition and operation of an emergency organization. Depending on the size and nature of the operation and the type of emergency, the functions identified here might or might not be performed by separate groups or individuals.

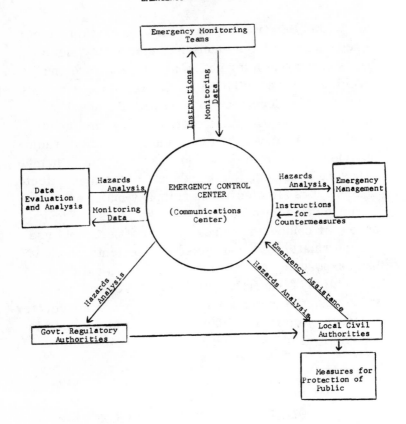

Figure 1

However, the functional requirements, as identified in the diagram, are usually present.

Emergency Control Center

The function of the emergency control center is to collect and transmit data, information, and instructions among the appropriate functioning units. The center should be staffed by individuals who have management authority (either directly or by delegation), well qualified in the field of radiation protection, and a detailed knowledge of the emergency plan. The staff provides initial instructions to appropriate operating units (such as emergency monitoring teams) and assures that incoming information is transmitted to those who need it. The center must be provided with suitable communications equipment, such as shortwave radios and telephones, and appropriate staff to operate the equipment. The importance of good communication cannot be overemphasized. As can be seen from the diagram, a breakdown in communications would jeopardize the functioning of the entire emergency organization.

Emergency Monitoring Teams

The function of the emergency monitoring teams is to conduct radiation surveys for the purpose of providing data about the radiation hazard. The teams should be staffed by personnel trained in monitoring techniques and emergency procedures. They should be provided with appropriate monitoring instruments, protective equipment, and communications equipment.

Data Evaluation and Analysis

The function of the data evaluation and analysis group is to collect the uninterpreted data provided by emergency monitoring teams, analyze it, and define the status of the emergency in terms which can be used by management and authorities as a basis for further actions. This group should be staffed by persons qualified in the field of radiation protection and might, as a practical matter, consist of the same persons who staff the emergency control center.

Emergency Management

Emergency management personnel are those who have authority to represent management in the event of an emergency. They make management decisions regarding emergency countermeasures during this period.

Local Civil Authorities

Local civil authorities, such as police, fire departments, and health organizations, are the first echelon of government with authority to implement measures for protection of the public in the vicinity of a licensed facility in the event of an accident. Since they are ordinarily the first source of outside assistance available in an emergency, civil officials should be briefed on the types of emergencies which may occur, the emergency plan, and the ways in which they might provide effective assistance. Civil authorities may take part in the emergency action at the request of the licensee or on their own volition as they deem necessary to fulfill their responsibility

to the public. Typically, they perform such functions
as controlling access to areas surrounding the plants,
help evacuate personnel, provide fire fighting capability, and medical assistance. State and Federal
assistance, such as might be provided by the AEC
Radiological Emergency Assistance teams, is usually
available. Federal and State organizations that have
regulatory authority over a licensed operation do not
usually become involved until the recovery phase
where they consult with licensee management about
plans for returning to normal operation, identifying
the cause of the emergency, and making changes in
operations where indicated to prevent reoccurrence
of the emergency.

Additional Functions

In addition to these major elements for management of an emergency situation, the licensee usually
provides additional in-house capabilities, such as
plant evacuation, fire fighting, medical assistance,
public relations, and area security, depending on the
nature of the operation and the types of accidents
which are credible.

Requirements for Emergency Monitoring

Returning attention to the role which monitoring
is intended to perform in an emergency, i.e., to provide information about the nature and magnitude of the
radiation hazard subsequent to an accident, it is useful to identify, as is done in Table I, the special
qualifications, requirements, or capabilities which
are necessary to accomplish these objectives when
developing an emergency plan. Training and

Table I

Special Requirements for Emergency
Monitoring Capability

Training	Instrumentation
1. Detailed knowledge of emergency procedures	1. Cover range of radiation anticipated in postulated emergencies
2. Ability to perform duties rapidly	2. Readily available
3. Ability to work under conditions of unusual physical and mental stress	3. Rugged
	4. Simple to operate
	5. Rapid measurement

instrumentation for operational monitoring are discussed in separate sessions of this Symposium and will not be covered in detail here except for any additional considerations related to emergency monitoring.

The type of training necessary to conduct emergency monitoring is roughly the same as that necessary for other types of operational monitoring. In addition to or knowledge of monitoring techniques, emergency monitoring personnel must be familiar with the details of the emergency procedures and be capable of operating under emergency conditions where a sense of urgency and chaos frequently prevails.

Time for gathering information is a crucial factor during emergencies. Therefore, those carrying out monitoring operations during the emergencies must be sufficiently proficient in their skills to perform their assigned duties rapidly.

There are few special characteristics for instruments by which they can be classified as emergency instruments as opposed to instruments used for other purposes. Generally, monitoring instruments designated for use during emergencies will be the same as those employed in normal operations. However, there may be a demand for special types of instruments to cope with postulated accidents, such as instruments capable of measuring abnormal levels of radiation or releases of radioactive material. Because of the nature of an emergency and the sense of urgency that prevails, special requirements for emergency monitoring equipment are that they should be readily available, rugged, simple to operate, and capable of making rapid measurements. To obtain some of these characteristics, it is ordinarily acceptable to sacrifice a degree of the measuring sensitivity that might be required for ordinary operation. Supplementary equipment necessary to implement emergency monitoring must be suitable for dealing with credible emergencies and must be compatible with the emergency procedure. There does not appear to be any specific inventory of instruments and equipment which would be appropriate for all emergencies that are credible within the nuclear industry without greatly overstocking for any given operation. Table II lists an equipment inventory for alpha-beta-gamma emergency monitoring used by the AEC Radiological Assistance teams. The equipment is simple and very

Table II

Equipment Inventory for Alpha-Beta-Gamma
Emergency Monitoring Kit used by AEC
Radiological Assistance Team

1 Alpha Scintillation Counter	1 Film Badge
	100 Foot Nylon Rope
1 GM Survey Meter	12 Radiation Signs
1 Jordan Survey Meter	1 Pencil
1 Pair Earphones	1 Notebook
2 Dosimeters (5 and 50R)	1 Flashlight and extra batteries
1 Dosimeter Charger	
1 Assault Mask	1 Roll Electric Tape
1 Pair Coveralls	1 Roll 2" Masking Tape
1 Pair Shoe Covers	2 Boxes Whatman Filter Paper
2 Pair Rubber Boots	
1 Head Cover	100 Cotton Tipped Swabs
1 Pair Canvas Gloves	1 Screw Driver
1 Pair Rubber Gloves	1 Pair Wire Cutters

easy to transport. Its utility, on the other hand, is rather narrow, being principally limited to determining levels of contamination and rather low levels of external radiation. The protective equipment in the kit is that which is ordinarily used where contamination, either airborne or surface, and low levels of radiation exist. It is obvious that many of the instruments used for emergency monitoring are the same as those used in daily operation and are capable of assessing a wide range of radiation hazards. On the other hand, such instruments require, in many instances, highly trained personnel to operate them effectively, a substantial monetary investment, and as a group are not easy to transport.

SUMMARY AND CONCLUSIONS

The safety standards employed in the nuclear industry do not eliminate the potential for an emergency arising but only reduce the probability of such an occurrence. Since this is the case, plans must be developed in advance to cope with emergencies which are credible in any given operation.

The most serious emergency should not serve as the sole basis for plan development. Rather, the plans should be designed to accommodate with greatest facility the more likely but less serious accidents. Emergency monitoring capability is an important part, but only a part, of emergency preparedness. It provides information about the nature and magnitude of the radiation hazard. Instruments used for emergency monitoring are frequently similar to those used in daily operational monitoring. In general, emergency monitoring instruments should be readily available, rugged, simple to operate and capable of making rapid measurements. Personnel who perform emergency monitoring should be well trained in instrument operation, have a detailed knowledge of the emergency procedure, and be capable of performing their duties under conditions of great stress.

EMERGENCY MONITORING OF AN INHALATION INCIDENT

Paul L. Ziemer and Robert R. Landolt
Bionucleonics Department, Purdue University
Lafayette, Indiana

INTRODUCTION

The purpose of this paper is not to deal with general monitoring procedures which may apply to all inhalation incidents, but rather to describe a specific inhalation incident and the health physics emergency procedures that were used. It is hoped that the event described will provide some useful insights so that others may benefit both from the successes and from the failures of this particular situation.

This discussion will be confined to a description of the incident, the immediate emergency procedures, the follow-up and decontamination, and the handling of press releases. Details on the biological aspects, including the long-term studies on the retention and excretion of the radioactive aerosol by the two persons involved have been described elsewhere.[1,2] We have not previously reported on the emergency monitoring aspects however, although the incident occurred about three years ago.

DESCRIPTION OF THE INCIDENT

The Sample

On August 30, 1965, an assistant professor of physics at Purdue University submitted application to the University health physics group requesting approval for a service irradiation of europium-153 from the Oak Ridge National Laboratory. The application called for the irradiation of Eu_2O_3 for 3 weeks at a flux of 2×10^{14} n/cm^2-sec. The sample was 2 mg of europium oxide enriched in stable europium-153 to 98.76% and supplied by the Isotopes Division of ORNL. Calculations indicated that such an irradiation would produce approximately 40 mCi of ^{154}Eu (Half-life: 16 years). The request was approved and submitted to Oak Ridge on September 30, 1965.

The irradiated sample was shipped from Oak Ridge on December 14, 1965, and arrived at Purdue on December 22 in a 525 pound shipping cask. At that time, one of us assisted in removing the source from the shipping container and transferring it to the isotope storage vault in Room B-26 of the physics building. At the time of the transfer, an unshielded reading made on the source indicated an exposure rate of 2.5 R/hr at one meter. (This value was recorded at the time as a matter of routine; later evaluation after the incident indicated that ^{154}Eu has a specific gamma constant of 7×10^{-1}R/hr/Ci at one meter. Hence the sample, if it were 40 mCi of ^{154}Eu, should have read only about 28 mR/hr at one meter.)

The Area

Room B-26 is a small laboratory having a floor size 8 ft by 10 ft (See Fig. 1). In the south wall is an isotope storage vault having 6 drawer type shelves with individual shielded doors. A hood and glove box are located along the east wall, with the workbench and sink on the west side. Entrance is from the north. The room is designed to have a net negative pressure with all air exhausting through a Kewaunee radiochemical hood with fiberglass filter and absolute filter. The hood runs continuously, pulling air into the room through a grill in the upper west wall. The floor was covered with smooth vinyl tile and the walls were coated with strippable paint. This room is one of a three room radioisotope suite which includes a low-level counting and teaching room, an intermediate level radiochemistry lab, and this higher level storage and sample preparation area. (See Fig. 1) A telephone had been installed in the corridor immediately outside the rooms to provide for emergency communications for all three laboratories.

Sequence of Events

The sequence of events leading up to and immediately following the incident insofar as we were able to later piece them together will now be described.

After entering the room, the two individuals were located as shown in Fig. 2. The professor removed the lead storage pig from the top left drawer of the vault, placed it on the bench top, and opened the lead pig to observe the size and shape of the quartz ampule prior to opening it. Normally, with a source of this type the quartz ampule is opened (by breaking) and the powder is dissolved in an appropriate reagent (acid in this case). At first he was hesitant to proceed because the ampule appeared to be of thin, pink-colored quartz rather than the dark brown quartz ampules which had

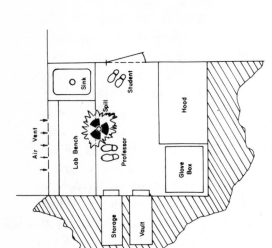

Fig. 2. Detail of High Level Radio-isotope Laboratory (Room B-26) Showing Approximate Positions of the Two Workers at the Time of the Incident.

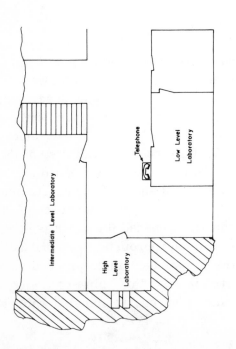

Fig. 1. Layout of the Three Lab Radioisotope Suite in the Basement of the Physics Building.

been associated with previous ampules of this type.
After a brief discussion with the student, he decided
to proceed, and removed the ampule from the lead
container with his gloved hand. In later statements,
he indicated that he tapped the vial against the lead
bricks which were sitting on the bench top to shake
the powder to one end of the sealed ampule in preparation for filing and breaking open. Before he could proceed further, and within a few seconds after the
tapping, the ampule exploded (or imploded) releasing
an europium oxide aerosol.

The professor immediately grabbed wet paper
toweling and picked up several large pieces of the
broken ampule from the floor. At this point he realized that his monitor was missing. (It was later determined that another staff member had removed the
monitor earlier that day and had taken it to the adjacent
laboratory. This fact had gone unnoticed up to that
point.) The professor asked the student to get the
monitor, and the student left the area. Instead of
checking the adjacent laboratory for the monitor, the
student went to get one from his own laboratory which
was, unfortunately, three floors up and on the far north
end of the building. He followed a route as indicated
in Fig. 3. When he reached his lab, he monitored
himself and discovered that his outer clothing was
contaminated. He removed only his sweater, which
seemed particularly hot, and then took the survey
meter and returned to the basement lab, this time
using a different route. The interval for this round
trip was about four minutes, during which time the
professor placed wet towels on the bench top, rolled
up the ampule fragments and towels in the absorbant
paper covering the bench and placed it all in the vault.

When the student returned he indicated that he had found himself to be contaminated. They attempted to check themselves further but found that the background in the lab was too high. Hence they proceeded to the adjacent laboratory and were able to monitor themselves. Realizing that they were both quite contaminated, they decided to call Health Physics. They removed their shoes prior to leaving the area. Interestingly, the professor took his shoes back to the original lab where the accident occurred, placed them inside the door, and locked the door to prevent entry. They then returned to the second floor laboratory to make the phone call to Health Physics, completely ignoring the telephone in the hall adjacent to the lab where the incident occurred. To make the situation even more complex, they used a third route, which included riding the freight elevator, to reach the upstairs lab (See Fig. 3).

INCIDENT TERMINATION AND EXPOSURE CONTROL

The call was received in the health physics office at 11:45 a.m. which was approximately 5 to 10 minutes after the incident occurred. The student gave the information that they had gotten the europium sample out to work with, it had exploded, and they were "slightly" contaminated but not hurt. We asked for their location and instructed them to stay there. We then proceeded to pick up our emergency kit. Being familiar with the sample in question, we expected air activity and took along a "Hi-Vol" sampler (which is not normally in our emergency kit).

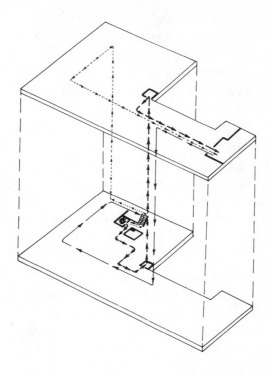

Fig. 3. Schematic showing basement floor and second floor of Purdue Physics Building. Spill occurred in basement room B-26 designated by the symbol ⬖. Initial route of student to second floor lab designated by short-dashed arrows ----►. Return route of student designated by long-dashed arrows————►. Final evacuation route indicated by heavy arrows ——►—►.

About two minutes after the first call, the student called back to tell us he had given us the wrong room number. With the corrected information, one of us (PLZ) and one of our graduate assistants in health physics went to the physics building.

The two health physics staff members arrived at the second floor laboratory about 11:55 a. m. or about 15 to 20 minutes after the incident and ten minutes after the first phone call. Although the phone information suggested that the contamination was slight, shoe covers, gloves, and respirators were donned before entering the laboratory where the contaminated individuals were waiting. At this point, the health physicists were still under the impression that the incident had occurred in this second floor laboratory.

It was clear, upon entering the room, that the contamination levels on the men were more than slight. They were literally covered from head to foot with activity. It would have been of great interest to make a detailed mapping of activity levels over their bodies, but expediency took precident over scientific aspirations and we immediately had them strip down to their shorts, collecting all clothes and personel articles in large plastic bags. Throughout this initial phase an air sample was collected in the room.

Simultaneously, the men were questioned about how the incident had occurred and where the spill was. It then became clear that it had taken place in the basement laboratory. One of us immediately went to the basement, wearing fresh shoe covers while approaching the hallway outside the basement lab. Background near the lab was too high to survey the hallway for tracking, so the area was roped off, the laboratory door was posted, and several smears were taken. A

quick check of other laboratories in the vicinity indicated that only one staff member was on duty (this was
lunch hour as well as Christmas vacation). He was
questioned briefly and stated that he had walked thru
the corridor a few minutes earlier. His shoes were
found to be slightly contaminated and hence were removed in favor of shoe covers prior to removing him
from the area.

An additional health physics technician who had
been collecting waste across campus when the emergency call came in, joined the group at this point and
took charge of counting the smears and checking for
tracking between the basement lab and the second
floor. At this time we were not aware of the original
trips made by the student to pick up a monitor nor did
he even recall this until a debriefing later in the day.
Hence, only the final evacuation route, which included
the elevator, was closely surveyed.

Meanwhile, in the second floor lab, the men had
completed stripping and had obtained nose swabs that
were highly contaminated. However, the external contamination on the hair, faces and forearms was so
great that it was difficult to verify whether the nose
swab was really picking up only skin contamination
from the face or if there had been significant deposition in the upper respiratory passages. The professor's head was reading 50 mR/hr at three inches
(read with a cutie pie) and the student's head was
reading about 20 mR/hr at five inches (maximum on
GMSM). Hence immediate decontamination of the head
and forearms was begun. This was done in the laboratory sink using cold water and mild detergent. A
large portion of the activity was removed by this
procedure and it was then readily apparent from direct

readings (over the sinuses and from nose wipes reading 20 mR/hr) that significant deposition had occurred.
It was decided at this point to place the men under
medical observation until an accessment of body burden and dose could be made. Because of Christmas
vacation and the fact that most students were away
from campus, the Student Health Center had only a
minimum staff on duty; thus it was necessary to use
a local hospital. We called our campus police and
requested assistance in transferring the men to the
hospital and asked them to alert the hospital and the
radiologist (who happens to serve part time in our own
health center as well.) The campus police were very
eager to assist, especially since they had just completed an emergency monitoring course a few weeks
prior to this. In fact, they not only provided assistance in transporting the men to the hospital, they
sent over several additional staff to assist in securing
the contaminated areas of the building. These men
remained on duty to assure that no one entered the
roped off areas.

    By the time we were ready to take the men to the
hospital, the health physics technicians had succeeded
in locating all the significant contamination along the
final evacuation route and had taken care of cleaning
up occasional hot spots in the halls, and on such spots
as the second floor button in the freight elevator.
They had also located all of the other people who were
in the building and had been near the area of the incident or had used the corridors or elevator along the
evacuation route. (Fortunately there were only a few
since school was not in session). Several low level
spots were found on shoes plus one contaminated fore-
finger where a graduate student had riden the elevator
and pushed the "Hot" second floor button.

By two o'clock (two hours after the incident) all areas were secure insofar as further spread of contamination was concerned. The fans in the basement of the building had been turned off to prevent possible spreading from the highly contaminated hallway just outside the lab where the incident occurred. The decision was made that the room where the incident occurred would not be entered even to access the extent of contamination inside until careful entry plans had been made. Thus the room was sealed off with tape and posted occordingly.

MEDICAL ASPECTS

Initial Handling

Upon reaching the hospital, the men underwent additional whole body decontamination in a restricted shower area in the hospital. We requested blood tests, collection of all excreta, and a lung scan on both men. Also we had periodic checks made with a portable survey meter on the nasal passages, lungs, and stomach. This provided a rapid estimation of the percentage of the material that was passing on to the gut and which would be rapidly eliminated. Both men stated that they were feeling fine. A mild laxative was administered at the hospital to hasten the elimination through the gut.

During the afternoon, we began, with our MD's to search for more information about europium, such as solubility data and biological and effective half life information, critical organ(s) and specific information on animal or human data. We even called a number of facilities around the country to determine if anyone had had any experience with europium.   The general answer was "no, but we will be interested in any information you might learn from the incident."

To assist our local doctors, who had very little experience in radiation emergencies, Dr. Eugene Saenger from Cincinnati was invited to provide medical consultation.   His assistance was invaluable, not only to the medical personnel, but to our health physics staff as well.   His broad experience with a variety of accidents helped our staff get this incident into a better perspective.

Estimation of Body Burdens

The fecal samples from the first forty-eight hours were counted, and based on a rough cross calibration with ^{137}Cs, an estimate of the amount of activity which cleared rapidly was obtained.   An estimate of 40 microcuries in the feces of the professor indicated that, if the old lung model were roughly correct, the body burden would reasonably be low.   Lung scans to estimate the lung burdens were made using the hospital's Picker Magnascanner.   A rough calibration was made with a ^{137}Cs jug phantom based on the specific gamma constants of ^{137}Cs and ^{154}Eu.

Using this crude method, it was estimated on December 30 that the individual with the highest lung burden had seven microcuries after the fecal clearance of the rapid components.   It is interesting to note that detailed whole body studies made over an extended period of time since the indicent indicated that the initial lung burden was about eleven microcuries. The key thing at the time was to get a good "ball-park" value for the lung burden so as to estimate dose. Based on the seven microcurie figure, it was clear that no therapeutic measures were required and arrangements were made to release the men from the hospital on December 30.

The long term retention and excretion data and the lung doses will not be discussed here since these have been reported elsewhere.[1,2]

DEBRIEFING

One difficulty in any accident is finding out what really happened. It was extremely difficult to obtain a clear picture of the incident while questioning the men during the first few minutes after the incident. There was the tension and confusion involved in attempting to do several urgent things at once: decontaminate the victims, prevent spread of addition contamination, secure the area where the spill occurred, locate tracked contamination, and arrange for medical support. These took immediate precidence over any attempt to enter into detailed questioning.

On the other hand, it is important to gain information as soon as possible while it is still fresh in the memory of those involved. Also, information could be uncovered that might have bearing on the further handling of the incident.

After the men had relaxed in their hospital room on the day of the incident, we interviewed them in more detail in an attempt to reconstruct details of the accident (times, sequence of events, etc.) This "debriefing" was beneficial. For example, it was through this detailed questioning that we first became aware of the fact that the student had followed two other routes to the second floor to obtain a monitor. Fortunately a

survey of these other routes indicated negligible tracking except for one stair case which we had discovered
previously anyway. But one might not always be so
fortunate, and the importance of attempting to gain such
information early cannot be over emphasized.

INFORMATION AND REPORTS

Notification of Government Agencies

Notification procedures were initiated within three
hours after the incident. This included immediate
notification of the AEC regional compliance office by
telephone and telegraph as required by 10 CFR 20[3],
and notification of the Indiana State Board of Health.

When we contacted the AEC, they advised that they
would send someone to observe and evaluate the situation. We were also advised to be prepared to issue a
press release. They indicated that it was their policy
to issue press releases on such incidents, but that we
could issue it directly provided that they approved
it first. We immediately alerted our Campus News
Bureau so that they could prepare to issue a release
at the appropriate time.

Information for News Media

Late on the evening of December 28, the day of the
incident, we prepared a memorandum explaining in
detail what had happened as far as we could evaluate it
at that time. Copies of this memo were delivered the
following morning to the University President and all
members of the Radiological Control Committee. The
information was sufficient so that the President could

issue a press release directly if he so desired. It was later confirmed that we should go ahead and prepare the press release ourselves. One of us (PLZ), together with the AEC representative who had arrived early that morning, and the chief of our News Bureau worked out a statement which was technically correct and which was journalistically acceptable. The statement was then phoned back to the AEC for review. They requested that we delete some of the material including the names of the individuals involved, the name of the nuclide and the activities involved. The resulting press release said essentially nothing very concrete. After this final draft was cleared by the President's office, the News Bureau prepared the press releases on their standard forms. These were sent to the local news media on the afternoon of the 29th, but by then it was too late to make the evening papers. Hence, no newspaper reports appeared until December 30, two days after the incident. This not only made the papers unhappy, but suspicious as well. As a result of the lack of information in the press release, the local papers dug out their own story. For example, the Lafayette Journal and Courier ran a picture of the Physics building under the caption "Contaminated Building." They also quoted at length the comments of one of the Deans who had only learned about the incident third hand. This included such statements as "the amount of contamination was so low that it hardly registered on the radioactive compass (sic) measuring instrument" and that the accident "involved no nuclear material, only mechanical radioactive particles."

The next day we contacted the local paper and arranged to have their reporter and photographer, come and see the accident scene and talk to our health

physics personnel. The reporter was shown the areas
where decontamination was in progress, and the sealed
lab where the incident occurred. He was briefed as to
the decontamination plans. By this time, we had already arranged for the release of the two men from the
hospital, and as everything seemed to be under control.
The papers did little more than to run a single follow
up story which was both informative and reassuring
to the readers.

The original statement was carried on the radio
and TV news at 5:30 p. m. on December 29th, about
one hour after the statement was released. The radio
stations had already learned the names of the two individuals by that time, so it really did not serve any
useful purpose to withhold the names originally. The
wire services picked up the story and brief articles
appeared in a number of papers, often under rather
humorous headings.

DECONTAMINATION

Decontamination of Adjacent Areas

Initial decontamination was directed toward cleanup of the corridor and laboratory adjacent to the room
where the incident occurred. Direct radiation exposure rates were not a problem, the maximum reading outside the spill area being only 16 mR/hr (see
Fig. 4). Tracking was not extensive beyond the hallway immediately outside the B-26 laboratory, and
boundaries defining contaminated areas were established
quite rapidly as shown in Fig. 4. The corridor and
the intermediate level lab (B-25) were zoned into a

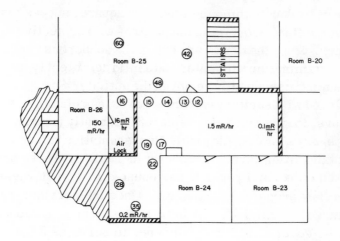

Fig. 4.   Restricted Area Following the Incident.
Stripped bars indicate locations of rope bar-
riers and of air lock.   Exposure rates indicated were measured 1 meter above floor level.
Numbered circles represent smear locations
where significant tracking had occurred (value
given in Table 1).

grid pattern of approximately 1 meter squares and then carefully decontaminated square by square, successively covering the decontaminated squares with protective paper. Since the floor was of smooth, nonporous vinyl, decontamination with water and a mild detergent type cleaning agent readily removed the activity. Sponge mops covered with sanitary napkins were used to clean the floors, the napkins being replaced frequently (usually for every square in the grid). Representative values of contamination levels are shown in Table 1. These are based on normal paper wipes counted in a windowless gas flow proportional counter. Once the corridor was cleaned, an air lock was built in the form of a wooden frame covered with polyethylene, to serve as a buffer zone and change area for later entrace into the lab where the spill occurred.

Decontamination of the High Level Laboratory

On December 30, four days after the incident, our health physics staff met with two representative from the Indiana State Board of Health* to plan for the initial lab surveys and evaluations. A list of equipment and supplies was drawn up and a plan of action formulated. On the evening of December 31, 1965, we entered the area for the initial surveys. This initial survey was to accomplish four objectives:

(1) Measure direct radiation levels
(2) Determine contamination levels
(3) Measure airborne activity

---

*We gratefully acknowledge the time and efforts of Henry C. Briggs and Hal Stocks for volunteering time and effort to assist in the early phases of contamination control.

Table 1.

Typical Contamination Levels from Tracking
Outside the Spill Area as Determined by
Floor Wipes.*

Wipe Location	cpm/$100cm^2$
12	6,600
13	3,700
14	22,000
15	10,000
16	21,000
17	3,205
19	10,500
22	15,725
28	3,150
35	332
42	6,900
48	3,350
60	13,000

* Wipes counted in a Nuclear Measurements PC-3A Gas
Flow Windowless Proportional Counter.

(4) Seal the package containing the broken vial
      and remove it from the area.

The two health physicists who made the initial entrance into room B-26 were suited-up in coveralls,
plastic pants, boots, gloves, plastic hats, and full-
face chemical oxygen supplies. Survey instruments
in protective plastic bags, portable low-volume air
samples, and materials for obtaining surface wipes
where taken into the room. Readings were verbally
relayed to a colleague outside the air lock who dictated
the results to a portable tape recorder.

Average background readings in the area were of
the order of 150 mR/hr. Direct readings on certain
spots on the floor read up to 5 R/hr beta plus gamma
read with a Juno type instrument. Smears were made
using sanitary napkins which were then sealed in plastic bags. These were read later by positioning them
10 cm from a portable survey meter in a nearby area
where background was normal. The smears all read
in the range of about 0.5 to 5 mR/hr at 10 cm. Air
activity was only about 0.05 MPC at that time.

The package containing the broken vial read
2 R/hr at contact. It was removed from the vault with
tongs and sealed in a plastic bag. It was passed out
thru the air-lock by a double bagging procedure and
removed from the area.

After the initial survey, which required less than
one-half hour, we withdrew and evaluated the situation
further. Based on the extremely high levels of surface
contamination, it was decided to coat the floor, lab
bench, and other surfaces with strippable paint to fix
the contamination for later removal. Hence the area
was reentered and the surfaces were coated with an

industrial strippable lacquer.* Later when the paint had dried sufficiently, it was found that it could be peeled off in sheets bringing large amounts of the activity with it. This worked quite well for the lab bench surfaces, but not too well for the floor. The paint solvents interacted with the vinyl to some extent, making it difficult to remove the paint and causing a discoloration of the vinyl.

It rapidly became evident that decontamination of the area would be a very slow process. Since our staff does not have sufficient personnel to drop everything and work at just one job, we began to think in terms of outside assistance.

The Radiological Control Committee approved this idea, and several commercial firms were contacted for bids. After the University business office gave final approval of the funds, final decontamination was contracted out. The decontamination can be summarized by saying that it consisted of vacuuming to remove all loose europium not tied down by the paint; removal of strippable paint; removal of the vinyl floor; cleaning the hood ducts and replacement of the prefilter and absolute filter, and scrubbing surfaces where necessary.

REEVALUATION OF SAMPLE ACTIVITY

It is of interest, to alert you to one aspect of this accident that must not be overlooked in any accident.

---

*Sherwin Williams Paint Co, Type M69 W1 Industrial Strippable Coating.

Namely, it turned out later that we were not really dealing with ^{154}Eu after all, at least not very much. This was initially suspected during the first few days after the accident and confirmed by about the second week. We initially took some of our smears and ran them in our gamma spectrometer. We were looking for ^{154}Eu plus some ^{152}Eu. Now both of these are fairly "messy" as far as having many photopeaks. Indeed, we found many peaks, some of which matched up fairly well with published spectra and some of which did not. Three separate events finally convinced us that what we really had was ^{156}Eu: (1) (1) Mr. Briggs, Indiana State Board of Health, continued to study the spectrum of one of the smears and identified some high energy peaks which could not have been from ^{152}Eu or ^{154}Eu. He had found that the activity on the smear was decaying away more rapidly than could be accounted for from the ^{154}Eu half life. (2) Our liquid scintillation whole body counting, which we initiated as soon as the men were released from the hospital showed daily decreases in body activity which could not be accounted for in the excreta, indicating rapid decay of a short-lived nuclide (3) Whole body crystal counting at Argonne by C. E. Miller confirmed that the predominant peaks were not those of ^{154}Eu. All evidence pointed toward ^{156}Eu. This would require significant triple neutron capture, but an examination of the cross section in going from ^{153}Eu to ^{154}Eu to ^{155}Eu to ^{156}Eu suggests that it certainly might be feasible. This was discussed with reactor personnel at both ANL and ORNL and although both groups at first said "impossible," they made some estimations and decided that a significant amount of ^{156}Eu could be formed. Later, detailed studies made by us using the decay of the sample to determine the relative abundance of 152, 154, 155 and 156 isotopes, coupled with activation calculations, indicated that the vial originally contained at the time of the exposure not forty millicuries of ^{154} Europium but

950 millicuries of ^{156}Europium
23 millicuries of ^{155}Europium
29 millicuries of ^{154}Europium
1.2 millicuries of ^{152}Europium

or over one curie of total activity.

The point to be made is, in any accident, be sure to verify that the material involved is what you think it is.

COST OF THE INCIDENT

It is difficult to access the overall cost of an incident, including all direct and indirect expenses. A reasonable evaluation of direct costs is feasible and was made for the incident described. These are listed below and include not only expenses directly paid out but also an estimate of the cost in salaries for the time devoted to the emergency by Purdue and State personnel.

Item	Cost
(1) Expendable supplies	$ 369.83
(2) Travel (Counting at Argone)	168.00
(3) Contaminated equipment disposed of	268.00
(4) Salary equivalent for Purdue and State personnel	2361.40

Item	Cost
(5) Europium sample lost	335.00
(6) Professional decontamination	2300.00
(7) Waste disposal	200.00
(8) New floor for B-26	50.00
(9) New filter for B-26	50.00
	$6102.23

It should be noted that these cost figures do not include
amounts paid by workmen's compensation for hospital-
ization and doctor's fees, amounts paid for the medical
consultant (this is handled by the AEC), nor any evaluation to account for the loss of time by the two victims.
Considering all factors, including indirect expenses,
it is probably reasonable to estimate the overall cost
of the incident to be between $7500-$10,000. Whether
or not one considers this costly is a matter of perspective. From the point of view of the University
type health physics operation, this incident was indeed
a costly one and represented a dollar value equivalent
to nearly 15% of our annual health physics budget.

REFERENCES

1. P. L. Ziemer, R. E. George, and W. V. Kessler,
    "The Uptake, Retention, and Excretion of Inhaled
    Curopium Oxide in Two Healthy Adult Males," Pro-
    ceedings of the First International Congress of
    Radiation Protection, Pergamon Press, Oxford
    (1968) pp 1199-1203.

2. R. E. George, "Whole Body Counting and Clearance Rate Study Following Accidental Europium Oxide Inhalation Exposure of Two Adult Male Subjects," Ph.D. Thesis, Purdue University, Lafayette, Indiana (1966).

3. Code of Federal Regulations, Title 10, Atomic Energy, Part 20.

AERIAL DETECTION AND RECOVERY
OF A COBALT-60 SOURCE
LOST IN INTERSTATE SHIPMENT

Harold E. Eskridge and John E. Hand,
EG & G, Inc., Las Vegas, Nevada

INTRODUCTION

This incident involved a 325 millicurie Cobalt -60 source which was being shipped by truck from Salt Lake City, Utah, to Houston, Texas, via Kansas City, Missouri. The source container was found to be upset and opened during a routine cargo inventory at the Kansas City terminal. The interstate carrier requested assistance from the AEC when he discovered that the source was missing.

The AEC sent a radiological assistance team which promptly determined that the source was not in the truck or the terminal. The AEC Division of Compliance verified that the source had been aboard the truck when it left Salt Lake City. Therefore, the source must have dropped off the truck somewhere between Salt Lake City and Kansas City, along a route of approximately 1100 road miles.

To rapidly survey the route taken by the express truck, the AEC called upon the Aerial Radiological Measuring Surveys (ARMS) airplane, operated for the AEC by EG & G, Las Vegas, Nevada. The route and rest stop locations were plotted on appropriate flight maps and a crew departed to begin the search at Salt Lake City.

LOCATION AND RECOVERY OF THE SOURCE

Arriving over the starting area, the aircraft descended to 400 feet above the terrain and began data collections along the route taken by the transport vehicle. No unusual radiation levels were observed during the first mission, covering the route between Salt Lake City and Cheyenne, Wyoming.

On the second mission, a sharp count rate peak, indicative of point source activity, was encountered soon after crossing the Missouri River at St. Joseph, Missouri. Spectral data confirmed that the high count rate was due to Cobalt -60. Additional passes were made to better define the source location on the embankment of the eastbound traffic lane. Figure 1 shows the route taken by the transport vehicle and the source location in relation to the town of St. Joseph, Missouri. Figure 2 shows the count rate trace recorded when passing over the source location.

The crew landed at the St. Joseph airport and obtained a rental vehicle and drove to the suspected source area. Using a portable scintillation rate-meter, the source was found two feet down the eastbound embankment. The closest residence was approximately 75 yards from the source location.

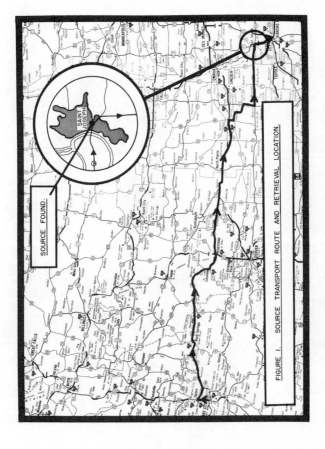

FIGURE 1.   SOURCE TRANSPORT ROUTE AND RETRIEVAL LOCATION.

Fig. 1.   Source Transport Route and Retrieval Location.

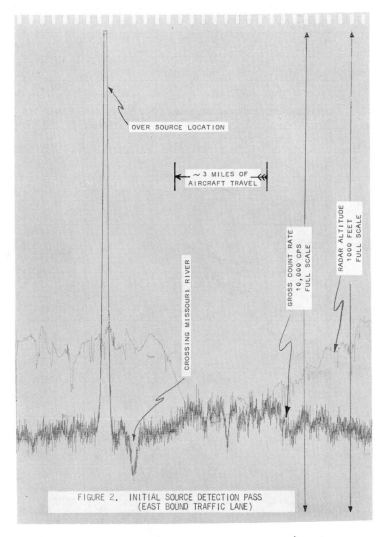

Fig. 2. Initial Source Detection Pass (East
Bound Traffic Lane).

The source was placed in a metal cylinder positioned in the center of a sand-filled wash tub for temporary shielding. This was accomplished in less than 48 hours after the request for assistance by ARMS.

ARMS INSTRUMENTATION AND CAPABILITY

The radiation detection and measurement systems in the ARMS aircraft consists of an array of fourteen 4" x 4" NaI(T1) detectors, a special purpose radiation computer, Doppler positioning equipment, single and multichannel analyzers, and various read-out equipment. Figure 3 is a functional block-diagram of the present instrumentation.

Figure 4 shows the detection capability of the system for point sources. A ten-fold increase in the minimum detectable activity is considered necessary to allow for variance in background and positioning in searching for a lost source.

Another application of the ARMS system is large area contamination surveys. The dose-rate levels are converted to levels at 3 feet above the terrain through experimentally determined conversion factors. Background and cosmic radiation contributions are subtracted. The ARMS aircraft is routinely used for large area surveys of power reactor sites.

CONCLUSIONS

As demonstrated by this incident, aerial surveying is an important tool for emergency monitoring, especially when large areas or distances are involved.

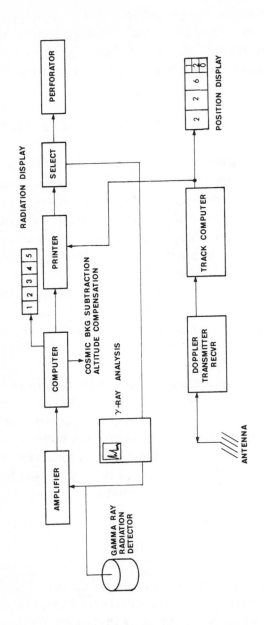

Fig. 3.   ARMS Instrumentation Functional Schematic.

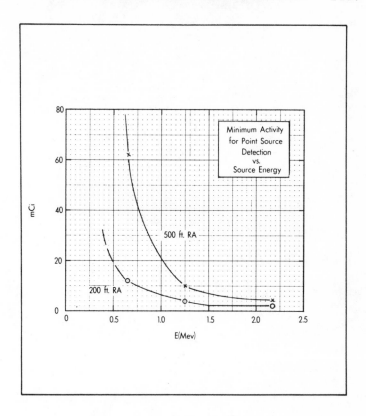

Figure 4.

Limitations are weather dependence and inability to detect beta-emitters and low energy gamma-emitters, unless the activity is airborne. Versatility of a survey aircraft may be extended by neutron and infrared detection, aerial photography, and air sampling capabilities.

FACILITY DECONTAMINATION FOLLOWING
A NUCLEAR ROCKET REACTOR TEST

John C. Gallimore and Joseph A. Mohrbacher
Pan American World Airways, Inc.
Aerospace Services Division
Nuclear Rocket Development Station Project
Jackass Flats, Nevada

I would like to discuss the health physics chal-
lenges and problems associated with the accomplishment of a sizeable decontamination effort following
testing of a nuclear rocket reactor at the Nuclear
Rocket Development Station (NRDS) in Nevada. This
station, an area of 140 square miles, is located 90
miles northwest of Las Vegas. This remote station
was established for the development and experimental
testing of nuclear rocket reactor and nuclear rocket
engine systems. To date, about 15 such experimental
units have been tested.

The first of one reactor series was tested on June
25, 1965. This test system is shown in Fig. 1. The
test system was operated at full design power and
temperature for approximately 10 minutes. Operation
was in good agreement with design predictions; however, during reactor shutdown, the liquid hydrogen
propellant supply in the test facility was unintentionally

1489

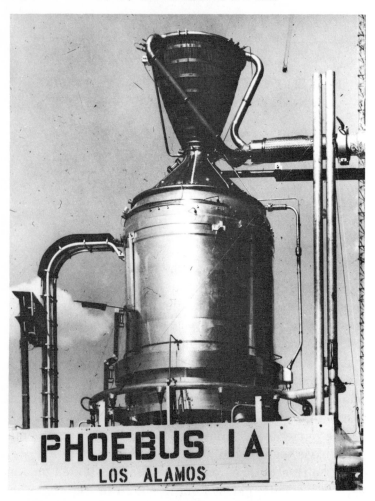

Fig. 1.   Phoebus 1A Nuclear Rocket Reactor
System--Designed and Constructed by the Los
Alamos Scientific Laboratory.

exhausted. This occurrence was not due to a reactor malfunction but rather to the malfunction of the liquid hydrogen storage dewar level guage which indicated a higher-than-actual content of propellant. This loss-of-coolant damage to the reactor resulted in the release of approximately 10 percent of the reactor core. It is estimated that at one hour post-shutdown 10^7 curies of fission product activity were deposited on the ground within the test facility. No significant fission product activity associated with this release was evident outside the test facility area. This is confirmed in a publication issued by the NUS Corporation (NUS 399).

Figure 2 shows a layout of the facility in which the test was accomplished. Following removal of the reactor, four days after the test, entry was made into the facility to establish radiation and contamination levels. The radiation conditions are shown in Fig. 3. Within the vicinity of the reactor pad, dose rates of 10 R/hr were encountered. No further penetration was accomplished at this time, as it was evident that much higher dose rates (estimated to 75 R/hr) would be encountered.

During the entry it was observed that an area of approximately 30,000 square feet--immediate surrounding the reactor position--was contaminated with fuel fragments from very small in size to about five inches in length. Fragments in excess of one inch in length were observed in concentrations up to one per ten square feet, with the smaller fragments present in much higher numbers.

Outside this highly contaminated area it was estimated that an additional 200,000 square feet were contaminated above the facility contamination guide of 2,000 d/m/ft^2.

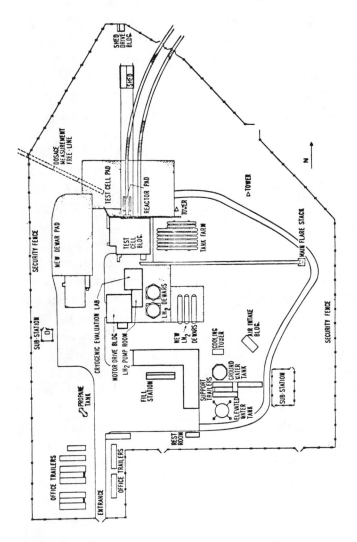

Fig. 2. Map of Test Cell "C".

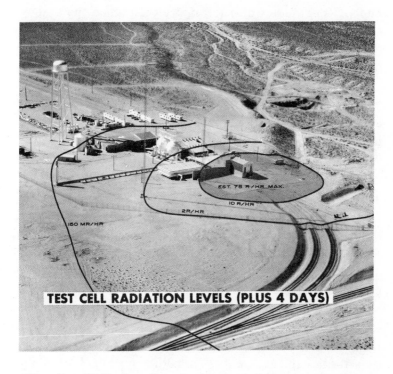

Fig. 3.   Radiation Levels in Test Cell at Four Days
Following Full Power Reactor Test.

A task force was convened to establish the objectives and a schedule for rehabilitation of the facility. Pan American World Airways, Inc. (Pan Am), the Support Services Contractor, was assigned the objective of decontamination of the Test Cell under certain ground rules of personnel exposure and damage to the facility.

Because of the excessively high dose rates which existed at this time, it was decided not to allow personnel into the facility until the maximum radiation level had decayed to about 10 R/hr. It was estimated that this would take three weeks. In the meantime the use of shielded or remotely operated equipment was attempted.

There existed on NRDS two vehicles—a shielded tank retriever and a shielded airplane tow vehicle. Attempts to utilize this equipment met with little success primarily because of poor maneuverability and possible damage to the facility; and their consideration was abandoned. A small remotely operated mobile manipulator was obtained and used for a very short time. The unit was extremely slow and could pick up only the large fragments. In addition to problems with its one dimensional television system, it crushed many of the smaller fragments under its tracks as it moved about in search of the large fragments.

Simultaneous with attempts to utilize the above equipment, a large vacuum system was evaluated for possible application. A system existed on site; and, could be utilized and was especially applicable to inaccessible locations. A unit was obtained and mounted on the rear of the shielded two vehicle. This unit is shown in Fig. 4.

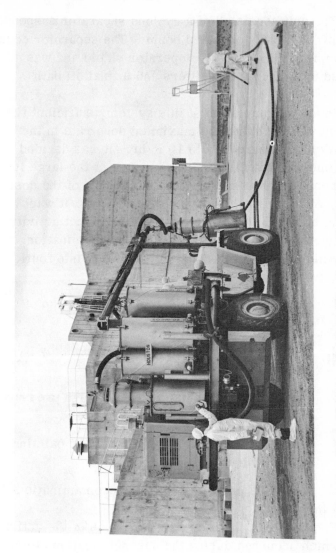

Fig. 4.   High Vacuum System Used for Collection of Reactor Core Debris.

The unit consisted of a cyclone separator suspended on a hydraulically operated boom.   The separator could be dumped from inside the operator shield and was backed up with four bag filters and a final oil bath filter.

Prior to completion of this system, sufficient time had elapsed such that the maximum dose rate in the Test Cell had decreased to 10 R/hr.   It was decided at this time to initiate the manned pickup of the large fuel fragments to effect an immediate lowering of the dose rate.   At this time, 24 days post-shutdown, it was estimated that 5,000 curies of fission product activity remained in the test facility.   The decontamination plan which had evolved could be separated into four phases:

1. Gross decontamination by manual pickup of the large fragments;

2. Collection of the remaining fragments by vacuuming and top soil removal;

3. Conventional decontamination by high pressure water and/or chemical treatment; and

4. Fixing the residual contamination by painting and other conventional methods.

Table 1 shows the chronology of the decontamination effort through release of the Test Cell.

Figures 5, 6, 7, 8, and 9 show some of the activities which occurred during the decontamination effort. Figure 10 shows the radiation condition of the Test Cell at the completion of the decontamination effort.

Rather than describe the operational details of the decontamination which are contained in a report

Table 1

Schedule of Decontamination Activities
Following Phoebus 1A

Activities	Post-Test Days
Phoebus 1A Full Power Test	0
Removal of Reactor from Facility	+4
Initiated Gross Decontamination	+24
Initiated Vacuuming	+31
Completed Gross Decontamination	+33
Completed Vacuuming	+36
Initiated Soil Removal	+37
Released the South Half of the Test Cell	+45
Released the Test Cell to Contractor Personnel	+59
Completion of Test Cell Decontamination	+63

(LA-3633-MS) issued by the Los Alamos Scientific Laboratory, I would like to discuss three areas which might be of interest to personnel involved in applied health physics activities. These areas are management and supervision of the effort, how we provided the large number of personnel required, and how we controlled their exposure. In addition, I would like to include what we learned about items which should be incorporated in the design of a test facility to facilitate decontamination.

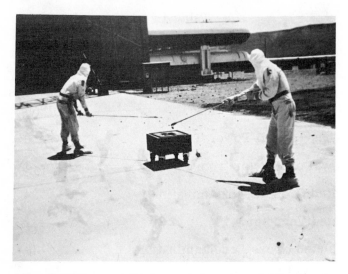

Fig. 5. Manned Pickup of Reactor Fuel Fragments.

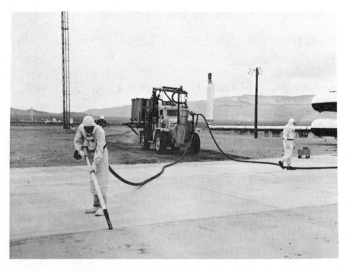

Fig. 6. Use of High Vacuum System in the Collection of Fuel Fragments.

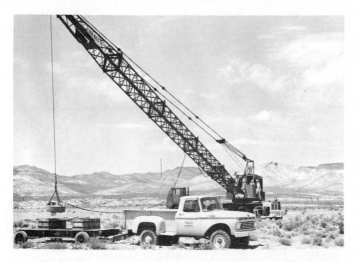

Fig. 7.   Pickup of Buckets containing
Fuel With an Electro-Magnet for transfer
to a Railroad Gondola.

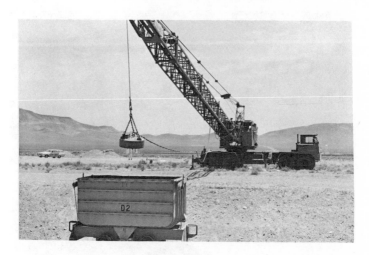

Fig. 8.   Transfer of Fuel to Railroad
Gondola.

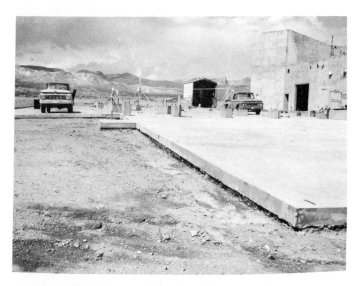

Fig. 9.   Decontamination By Soil Removal.

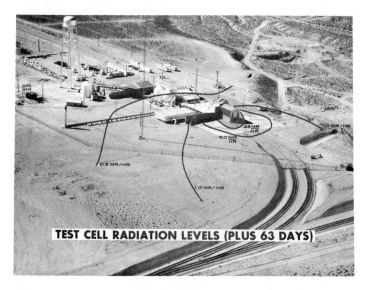

Fig. 10.   Radiation Levels in the Test Facility
at Completion of Decontamination.

MANAGEMENT AND SUPERVISION

One of the accomplishments which contributed significantly to the success of the effort was a formulation of a decontamination plan during the initial deliberations of the task force. This plan, in addition to setting up the ground rules, defining responsibilities, established the decontamination objectives and the schedule by which they were to be accomplished. An example of one complication which the plan resolved was test cell modifications by off-site contractor personnel which were to be accomplished prior to receiving the next test article. This contract, for economic reasons, resulted in the necessity to decontaminate the contractor area to off-site release levels. By decontaminating to these levels, the contractor would not be delayed by having to use protective clothing or otherwise, comply with radiation control procedures. With this and other contingencies resolved by the plan, realistic objectives and schedules were known from the outset; and targets or milestones could be established toward which all efforts could be directed.

With all objectives clearly stated, detailed decontamination procedures were prepared in advance, allowing time for material and equipment acquisition, procedural dry runs, training, and advance scheduling of activities and personnel.

With Pan Am assigned the decontamination responsibility, it was necessary to establish the management framework within Pan Am by which this work could be accomplished. This also proved to be a significant contribution to the success of the decontamination effort. First of all, because of the levels to which decontamination had to be performed and the urgency involved, it was necessary to give the operation "top priority." One individual was assigned the overall responsibility for management and conduct of the effort. Authority was given this individual to cross departmental lines and responsibilities as necessary to effect this decontamination. This was especially important in that this individual could select line supervision of his choice to direct the actual decontamination. Selection and training of line supervision to direct the actual work was, in our opinion, responsible for the excellent productivity which we obtained from the decontamination personnel.

Lack of assigning adequate supervision to the operation was evident near the end of the effort. Fatigue and radiation exposure resulted in reduced efficiency and effectiveness in two key personnel assigned to the operation. Additional supervision, trained and current with the operations, should have been available to relieve these personnel without affecting continuity of the operations.

SELECTION OF PERSONNEL

In performing the decontamination effort it was necessary to assemble a large group of personnel; and, because of the exposure which would be involved, it was necessary to utilize personnel who did not receive radiation exposure in the normal course of their work. Approximately 400 personnel from various crafts were available, which included: carpenters, plumbers, painters, pipefitters, supply clerks, welders, electricians, heavy equipment operators, cryogenic technicians, janitors, and laborers. Many of these personnel had worked within a controlled radiation area, however, never with the radiation and contamination levels which existed within the test facility. Therefore, it was necessary to give these personnel training in decontamination and radiation safety principles.

This program was established and given in a 3-hour period of intensive lecturing and demonstrations. The training was given well in advance of the individual's assignment to the decontamination effort with a refresher discussion provided immediately prior to his entering the test facility. This program included:

— Radiation/Contamination Levels and Required Precautions.

— Radiation Exposure Criteria.

— Use of Anti-Contamination Clothing.

— Use and Care of Respiratory Protective Equipment.

— Use and Care of Film Badge and Pocket Dosimeters.

— Contamination and Contamination Control, and

— Decontamination Procedures.

An employee with a physical condition which might affect his safety and performance was evaluated by the Medical Department prior to his assignment.

Logistics of scheduling and transporting of these personnel to the decontamination check station such that lost time was minimized and operational continuity maintained, proved to be a very serious problem. Because it was essential that other support continue, no single shop could be stripped of personnel for the decontamination program. An individual was established with the sole responsibility of scheduling the required personnel with emphasis on minimum interruption of activities in the various disciplines. Only after establishing this procedure was this critical operation satisfactorily accomplished. This permitted the decontamination supervisor to concentrate on the task to be performed without concern as to whether trained personnel would appear or not.

EXPOSURE CONTROL

Exposure control was based on the philosophy of uniform distribution of exposure among the participants. An administrative guide of 1R was established for the initial participation. All exposures in excess of this guide required approval at the Project Manager level. This approval did create delays, as it was necessary on a number of occasions to exchange personnel when only a few more mR exposure was required to complete an operation. The authority for exposure control should have remained with those personnel directly responsible for the decontamination.

Approximately 200 Pan Am personnel participated directly in the decontamination effort, accumulating a total exposure of just over 150R with an average of about . 7R.

Direct reading dosimeters were used to maintain current exposure estimates. Exposure was based primarily on time and dose rate. However, because of the many locally high dose rates, a Radiation Monitor was assigned to each group of decontamination personnel to frequently check the dosimeter readings to assure that dose guides were not exceeded. Film badges were exchanged when the accumulated dose exceeded an estimate of .15R.

Exposure control regarding airborne radioactivity was accomplished utilizing full face masks. Although cross-contamination was eminent on windy days, air samples taken during the decontamination effort rarely indicated re-suspension of activity. However, because particle inhalation and the possibility of having a particulate deposited in the eye could not be ruled out, full face masks were worn during operations which could produce local airborne contamination on windy days.

FACILITY DESIGN

In order to reduce the decontamination time and radiation exposure to a minimum, careful consideration must be given to "ease of decontamination" in the original design of a facility. These considerations are usually given and solutions incorporated in the design; however, they are often deleted or traded for more critical items because of budget problems. These considerations are especially important in a research and development test facility where contamination is probable and the schedule is critical. The following list presents a number of items which, from our experience, should be incorporated in the design of such a facility:

— Minimum inaccessible locations where contamination could accumulate. If outside piping and open structures are necessary, they should be arranged such that personnel and equipment can gain easy access.

— If practical, all outside areas within the facility should be concreted. If concrete is not practical, soil or gravel should be contoured to eliminate fills and slopes.

— Concrete areas, including building roofs, should be properly sloped, curbed, and drained. Drains should be checked frequently to assure proper operation. Building roofs should be kept clear and not contain piping and equipment which would not only accumulate contamination but interfere with decontamination.

— All concrete expansion joints should be sealed and the concrete area painted.

— An abundant number of fire hydrants above that normally required in the fire protection system, strategically placed, should exist.

— All areas of the facility should be equipped with adequate lighting, permitting a decontamination effort to continue into the night.

— All outside electrical equipment and other critical items should be waterproofed. This would permit the use of high pressure water—the most economical decontaminating agent.

— All building floors should be properly sloped and drained. In addition, sufficient space should be allowed under the equipment for cleaning. If at all possible, waterproofing of electrical and sensitive equipment should be accomplished inside the buildings.

— All underground plumbing and electrical systems should be precisely documented in engineering drawings.

The preceding items apply primarily to a type of facility in which our decontamination effort was acomplished. However, many of them would be applicable to any type facility where radioactive material is utilized.

Health Physics personnel should make every effort to insure that the Design Engineer includes "ease of decontamination" in his facility design; and, if for some reason this cannot be accomplished, management should be advised of the possible consequences.

EMERGENCY DECONTAMINATION FACILITIES

G. R. Yesberger
U. S. Atomic Energy Commission
Richland Operations Office
Richland, Washington

ABSTRACT

The "SL-1" criticality accident provided an opportunity for atomic energy installations to examine their capabilities and facilities for handling such an accident. It became apparent to Hanford that we were unprepared for such an occurrence and corrective measures were initiated.

Although a radio-surgery facility was completed at Hanford, emergency decontamination facilities must be available in close proximity to work sites to provide prompt gross decontamination of accident patients emanating high level gamma radiation. The basement of a laboratory area complex and the automotive garages in our production areas have been equipped at minimum expense to provide such gross decontamination services, yet the primary use of the facility remains unaffected.

The use of the decontamination facilities has not been required to date but they are maintained in a state of readiness.

G. R. YESBERGER

INTRODUCTION

A radiation accident has been defined by Dr. E. L. Saenger[1] as an unforeseen occurrence, either actual or suspected, involving exposure of or contamination on or within humans and the environment by ionizing radiation.

In spite of the many safety measures and precautions which are taken, radiation accidents can and will continue to take place within the nuclear industry whether we work in a university, small radio-chemical plant or at a major Atomic Energy Commission site. We should all have plans for coping with and minimizing the consequences of these accidents. Many of these radiation accidents will involve contamination of personnel and thus facilities of varying complexity may be required for decontamination purposes. The purpose of this presentation is to describe in a very brief manner the various types of personnel emergency decontamination facilities which are or could be used at Hanford. The medical aspects, instrumentation, and dosimetry considerations are not treated in this discussion.

LABORATORY DECONTAMINATION FACILITIES

We are fortunate that in a great majority of the personnel contamination cases there are no injuries or breaks in the skin and decontamination may be accomplished with little or no difficulty at or near the work location. A medical case involving radioactive contaminants will usually require some degree of decontamination before the patient is transported to the medical facility or when necessary, to the community hospital. In the case of gross body contamination, the prompt removal of clothing and wash-down or showering of the worker may be necessary. Immediate flushing with water may be required in the event of an open wound or eye contamination or when strong acids or bases are present. Decontamination should be accomplished as soon as possible, but care should be exercised so that the personnel involved are not further contaminated during the decontamination process. The emergency medical care of the patient, such as control of breathing or bleeding, is of prime consideration and the decontamination or prevention of spread of contamination of secondary importance.

A typical example of a normal laboratory type decontamination facility is noted in Fig. 1. A saturated potassium permanganate solution is being used to remove some plutonium contamination from a worker's finger. It is important that written procedures be available which specify decontamination methods and agents to be employed. The procedures should consider the various types of contamination which may be encountered, such as localized skin contamination, particle contamination, general body contamination, and hair, eye, nose or mouth contamination. The chemical and physical state of the contaminant should be known as well as the radionuclide(s) involved. It is recommended that health physics personnel maintain close liaison with and obtain approval of their medical organization insofar as decontamination agents and procedures to be followed. One should always be alert as to the condition of the skin being contaminated in order that it is not injured in the decontamination process. We should always look for skin breaks, punctures, burns, etc. in that serious internal exposures of personnel may result if radioactive contaminants are allowed to enter the body through these routes.

The standard portable decontamination kit[2] used at Hanford is noted in Fig. 2. Each facility should

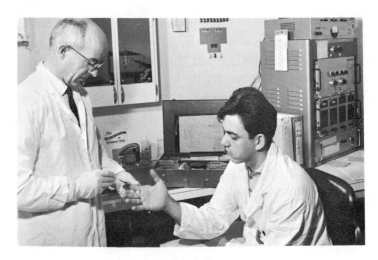

Figure 1.
A Laboratory-Type Decontamination Facility

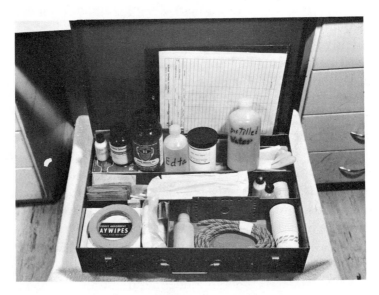

Figure 2.
The Hanford Decontamination Kit

have ready access to such kits which contain materials expressly used for personnel decontamination. These supplies should be inventoried on a regular established basis. A lead spotting shield is a practical item which should be included in every kit for delineation of local contamination.

RADIOSURGERY FACILITY

Following the SL-1 criticality accident, plans were made for the construction of an emergency decontamination or radiosurgery facility at Hanford. Such a facility was completed adjacent to our community hospital last year and is operated by the Hanford Environmental Health Foundation for the AEC.[3] This facility is located about 8 miles from our laboratory area and 30 miles from our large production reactors and separations plants. In addition to fulfilling its primary objective of facilitating treatment or surgery on highly contaminated patients, the facility was constructed in order to perform research and development in such areas as improved methods, technology, and cell design. The shielding and patient handling equipment is noted in Fig. 3.

If needed, the patient receives a general body wash and scrub-down in the shielded body wash upon arrival to remove loose contamination. All liquid waste from this cell and the shielded surgical table drains into a 500 gallon holding tank. The patient is then placed on a mesh type litter, suspended by a monorail, where he is moved to the shielded surgical table which provides 4" of steel shielding for the medical and health physics staff. Lead head and neck shields with lead glass viewing ports are provided for the surgeon and attending personnel. The shielding was designed to provide a nimimum reduction factor of about 50 for all anticipated contamination

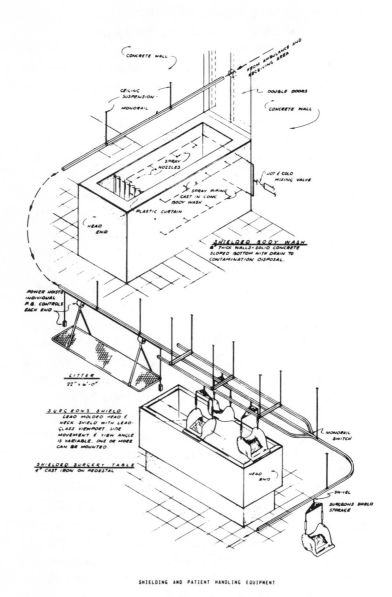

SHIELDING AND PATIENT HANDLING EQUIPMENT

Figure 3.
Handord Decontamination and Radiosurgery Facility.

disposal features of cell design provides for air and
liquid waste to exit through the base of the unit.   The
floor plan of the facility is shown in Fig. 4.   Two cells
have been completed and space made available for two
future additional cells.   The ventilation system provides for high efficiency filtration of all air leaving
the facility.   Shielded containers are provided for the
storage of solid waste.   A room is provided for storage
of health physics instrumentation and decontamination
supplies.   Air sampling stations are also provided
throughout the facility.   The exterior of the building
showing the ambulance entrance is noted in Fig. 5.
The total building comprises some 3,185 square feet.
A photo of the interior of the building showing the two
in-place surgical cells is noted in Fig. 6.   A close-up
of the radiosurgery cell noting how attendants would
provide medical or surgical care of a patient is noted
in Fig. 7.

EMERGENCY DECONTAMINATION

It is realized that emergency surgery or decontamination of a patient highly contaminated with gamma
emitting radionuclides may be required before a patient
could be transported to the radiosurgery facility.
Because of this, and as a measure to provide some
type of backup for the radiosurgery facility, standby
equipment for an emergency decontamination facility
is available in each of our major plant areas.

Figure 8 notes the emergency decontamination
equipment and temporary shielding which is provided
in one of the Battelle Northwest Laboratory buildings.
Running hot and cold water is available at each site.
Other equipment which is stored at each site include
a portable lead glass shield, plastic bags, lead bricks,
scrub brush, detergents, etc.   Emergency medical
and surgical supplies are maintained at each major

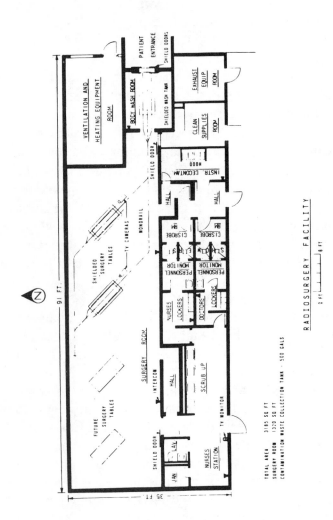

RADIOSURGERY FACILITY

TOTAL AREA   3185 SQ FT
SURGERY ROOM   1320 SQ FT
CONTAMINATION WASTE COLLECTION TANK — 500 GALS

Figure 4.

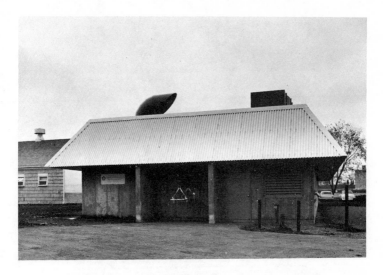

Figure 5.
Exterior of the Radiosurgery Facility.

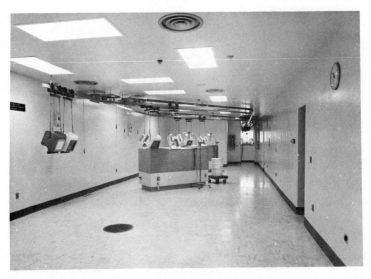

Figure 6.
Radiosurgery facility interior.

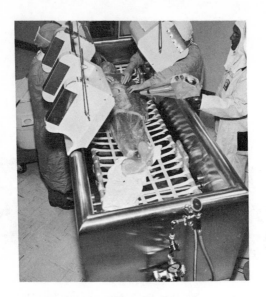

Figure 7.
The Radiosurgical cell.

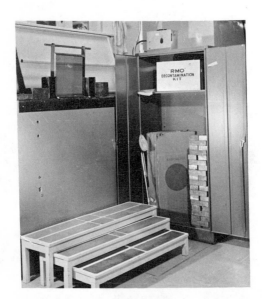

Figure 8.
Emergency decontamination equipment and temporary
shielding

site by our medical organization. Step stools of various
heights are provided at this location in order to
accommodate decontamination or medical personnel.
Figure 9 notes how a grease pit in our plant garages

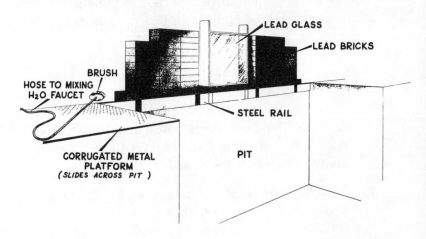

EMERGENCY RADIO-SURGERY
LEAD BRICK AND LEAD GLASS SHIELD ARRANGEMENT

Figure 9.

may be used to provide this type of decontamination or
temporary radiosurgery facility. Supplies identical
to those as shown in the previous slide are stored in
cabinets in each of our outer area garages. Although
we have never had an occasion to use these emergency
decontamination facilities, we do feel that they would
be of great value in the event of a major plant accident
involving high level contamination of personnel.

CONCLUSION

Emergency plans should be available for coping and minimizing the effects of all anticipated contamination events. Drills should be conducted on a periodic basis to test the effectiveness of these plans. Personnel decontamination facilities of varying complexity will be required depending on types and quantities of radionuclides handled. Although I don't feel it necessary that a Hanford-type radiosurgery unit be constructed at every location, I would recommend that an examination of your facilities be made to determine where and how the decontamination of a high contaminated person may be performed should you ever be faced with this possibility.

REFERENCES

1. E. L. Saenger, Medical Aspects of Radiation Accidents; A Handbook for Physicians, Health Physicists and Industrial Hygienists. U. S. Government Printing Office, 1963.

2. Battelle Northwest - Procedures for Radiation Monitoring, Pages 4-1 through 4-10 of BNWL-MA-7, February 1, 1968.

3. C. M. Unruh, H. V. Larson, and P. A. Fuqua, "The Hanford Radiosurgery Facility," June 1968.

A PLAN FOR EMERGENCIES

G. T. Lonergan
Argonne National Laboratory*
Argonne, Illinois

ABSTRACT

Argonne National Laboratory's organization for
handling emergencies is designed to provide positive
action directed at the protection of personnel and the
minimization of property damage. The general plan
for handling emergencies places the responsibility
for evaluation and control of incidents in the hands of
the local Area Emergency Supervisor. Responsibilities of both the local Area Emergency Supervisors and
the Laboratory Emergency Coordinator are outlined.
Notification of emergency response units and
emergency supervisors is accomplished through the
utilization of the Group Alerting System. Initial
notification of a criticality is tied into the Group
Alerting System. A summary of responsibilities of
normally responding forces is presented. Preplanned

*Work performed under the auspices of the United
States Atomic Energy Commission.

actions of various response groups for specific types
of emergencies are outlined.

INTRODUCTION

The plan for emergencies discussed in this paper
pertains only to Argonne National Laboratory's
Argonne, Illinois site, where approximately 5500
individuals are employed. The Illinois site occupies
3700 acres in DuPage County and is located approximately twenty-seven miles southwest of downtown
Chicago, Illinois.

The Laboratory carries on a broad program of
research in the areas of reactor sciences, physical
sciences and life sciences.[1] The physical facilities
are composed of one-hundred-and-seventy-three (173)
numbered buildings and/or structures which comprise
3,366,551 square feet of floor space. As in any
facility of this type a definite effort is directed toward
the prevention of emergencies. The size of this effort
in no way diminishes the necessity of advance planning
for emergencies. Advance planning allows time for
consideration of alternatives. Planning aimed at the
prevention and minimization of emergencies is the
responsibility of all groups at Argonne.

THE EMERGENCY PLAN

The basic plan establishes the emergency force
structure and describes the positions within the
structure. It defines responsibilities and provides a
framework for general and specific plans. The plan

is both flexible and efficient.   The plan provides for informed evaluation at the scene of the emergency and utilization of the emergency response capabilities in the manner and to the degree necessary to control the situation.   ANL emergency planning is designed first to protect lives and second to protect property.

The following guidelines are provided Laboratory personnel for the implementation of the two purposes for emergency planning.[2]

Lives of Laboratory personnel, visitors and the public will be protected; an emergency will be contained in the most limited area possible; equipment and facilities will be protected to the greatest extent possible; all possible salvage action will be taken; action will be taken to secure the affected area or facilities; and, areas or facilities will be turned over to the appropriate services for restoration at the earliest opportunity.

TYPES OF EMERGENCIES

It is appropriate at this point to define the two phases of emergencies as the terms are used at Argonne.   The initial phase begins with the report of the emergency, usually a telephone call to extension "13" and includes alerting, initial response and controlling activities at the scene by those emergency response units which respond to the first alert.   This is a general description of the DIAL 13 procedure, a mechanism by which any individual may report what he may consider to be an emergency.   A guideline as to what can be considered an emergency is provided to all employees: "If immediate action is needed to prevent injury or property damage, or if a particular incident cannot be handled with one routine telephone call, the situation is an emergency."[2] This is a very broad and inclusive definition; however, it is so intentionally and in line with the Laboratory's preference of having its employees err on the side of safety with respect to reporting occurrences than to allow a serious situation to develop because an individual delayed too long or failed to report a situation which might require emergency assistance. All emergencies are considered to be DIAL 13 emergencies unless declared a Major Emergency by an Area Emergency Supervisor. The guidelines used by Area Emergency Supervisors in determining whether or not a DIAL 13 emergency is to be classified as a Major Emergency are as follows:[2]

Any emergency or occurrence which involves one or more buildings or areas; and,

any emergency or occurrence which requires support beyond those capabilities and services of those groups which respond under the DIAL 13 procedure.

EMERGENCY FORCE STRUCTURE, POSITIONS AND RESPONSIBILITIES

The structure of the emergency organization is built around the Emergency Coordinator and those individuals designated as the Area Emergency Supervisors and their alternates. Laboratory-wide emergency response capabilities are provided by the organizations listed in Fig. 1.[2]

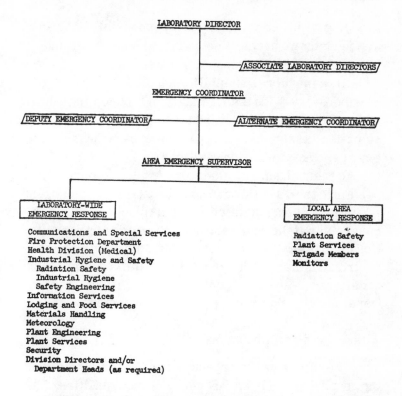

Fig. 1.   ANL Emergency Force Structure.

The heads of the Laboratory-wide emergency response organizations act in the capacity of a special staff
to the Emergency Coordinator during major emergencies.

Emergency Coordinator

The Emergency Plan provides an individual at the
top of its organization who is able to communicate with and
for management about and during emergencies. This individual is the Emergency Coordinator. He is responsible
for developing the overall plan. He assures the economical
application of emergency forces, personnel and equipment

in coping with emergencies. His responsibilities can be
divided into two areas: General Responsibilities and
Major Emergency Responsibilities.

His general responsibilities include the preparation
of Laboratory-wide emergency plans, becoming familiar
with individual unit plans and insuring their effectiveness,
selection, assignment of and training individuals in key
emergency organization positions.

In event of a major emergency, his responsibilities
pertain to the direction and coordination of all emergency
activities. He consults with the pertinent Area Emergency
Supervisor at the scene and obtains advice and consultation from his emergency force staff. He establishes a
control command post from which he initiates appropriate
orders regarding emergency communications, evacua-
tions, facility shutdown, public announcements, etc.

Alternate Emergency Coodinator

The Alternate Emergency Coordinator carries out
the general and major emergency responsibilities of the
Emergency Coordinator in the absence of the Emergency
Coordinator.

Deputy and Alternate Deputy Emergency Coordinator

Much of the detail and duties, e.g., assessing skills
and limitations of the overall emergency response capability is located in the general responsibilities of the
Deputy Emergency Coordinator and Alternate Deputy
Emergency Coordinator positions. The individuals assigned to these positions are required to know and review
the various detailed plans of emergency units and make
proposals necessary to assure integration of individual
unit plans with the overall emergency plan. The Deputy
and Alternate Deputy Emergency Coordinator maintain

liaison with appropriate Federal, state and local organizations to insure compatability of the Laboratory's emergency plans with those of the contacted organizations. All emergency drills are coordinated by the Deputy and Alternate Deputy. This includes reviews and critiques of drills or other exercises and modification of procedures as required. They are, in cooperation with Division Directors, responsible for the selection and assignment of individual Area Emergency Supervisors. They also serve as a staff advisor to the Emergency Coordinator during major emergencies.

Area Emergency Supervisor
and Alternate Area Emergency Supervisor

Seventy-one (71) individuals are assigned as **Area Emergency Supervisors** and/or Alternate Area Emergency Supervisors. Each Area Emergency Supervisor and his alternate are assigned responsibilities for a specific building or area.

Just as the Emergency Coordinator is responsible for the overall emergency plan and capabilities, the Area Emergency Supervisor is responsible for the emergency plan and capabilities within the limits of the particular area or building to which he is assigned. The Area Emergency Supervisor is an extension of the Emergency Coordinator. He too communicates with and for the management in the area to which he is assigned. He is also the spokesman for the Emergency Coordinator in that area. He is aware of and involved in the day-to-day and planned operations, construction and modification of facilities in his area of assignment. In short he is an individual who can get things done in planning for the prevention of emergencies,

and the successful handling of incidents once they
occur.

The Area Emergency Supervisor is responsible
for the control, direction and coordination of actions
taken at the site of the occurrence. However, he remains under the operational control of the Emergency
Coordinator during emergency operations.

The Area Emergency Supervisor must become
thoroughly familiar with situations and conditions which
could be classified as potential emergencies. He like
the Emergency Coordinator must prepare or cause to
be prepared adequate plans for coping with emergencies which may occur in his area, and insure the compatability of such plans with the overall plan. The
Area Emergency Supervisor must be thoroughly
familiar with facility services in his area, i.e., power,
water, ventilation, scientific and emergency equipment, switches, valves and other controls. He plans
and conducts training of building emergency force
personnel which he recruits for a particular emergency position.

During an emergency, he reports to the location
of the incident, establishes an emergency control
point and makes an overall evaluation of the situation.
He directs evacuation as necessary and mobilizes
brigade personnel as required. If he does not classify
the incident as a major emergency, he directs and
coordinates all emergency control activity at the scene.
Additional support and services are made available
from the Laboratory-wide response groups and pertinent divisions upon his request to the Emergency
Coordinator in situations requiring such assistance,
i.e., major emergency.

Upon gaining control of the situation, he alone will declare the termination of emergency response group actions by announcing the ALL CLEAR by means of the DIAL 13 procedure. For those emergencies which result in damage or personal injury, he will hold an incident review meeting and provide a report to the Emergency Coordinator.

Selection and Assignment

The position of Emergency Coordinator and the positions of the Area Emergency Supervisors and their designated alternates are filled by individuals who accept the responsibilities of their particular emergency position in addition to their regular full-time duties.

As is the case with any assignment which is considered as an additional duty and involving a relatively large number of individuals, transfers, relocation, terminations, etc. requires from time to time the designation of new or replacement Area Emergency Supervisors and/or Alternates. The maintenance of the roster of individuals assigned as Area Emergency Supervisors is the responsibility of the Emergency Coordinator. However, the actual selection lies within the duties of the Deputy Emergency Coordinator and the Division Directors. Turnover in personnel assigned to these positions is minimized by the selection of individuals who are thoroughly versed in the facilities, equipment, hazards and personnel capabilities in the area to which they are assigned. The individual who fits these requirements is usually a long-term employee with considerable experience in positions of responsibility.

Division Directors and Department Heads

No emergency organization could properly function without a communication link between the occupants of the buildings, or areas and the emergency
organization. This communication and supervisory
link is supplied by the Division Directors or Department Heads. The major responsibility of the Division Director or Department Head is constant vigi-
lance and anticipation of potential emergency situations
existing in his particular area or which may result
from his division's operations. He is responsible
for establishing procedures to avoid such emergencies
and for handling those that do occur.

Security Division Lieutenant

Certain organizations within the Emergency
Force Structure have an around-the-clock capability.
They are the Fire Protection Department, Security
Division, Plant Services, Industrial Hygiene and
Safety—Radiation Safety.

The positions of Emergency Coordinator and
Area Emergency Supervisor and their designated
alternates are normally filled by individuals who are
not available at the site twenty-four hours a day.
During other than normal working hours, the duties
of the Emergency Coordinator and the Area Emergency
Supervisor are assumed by the Security Division
Lieutenant on duty until properly relieved by the
Emergency Coordinator or the appropriate Area
Emergency Supervisor.

Emergency Brigades[2]

Emergency brigades are made up of individuals who have excellent knowledge of specific work areas and the physical capability to provide effective assistance in emergency situations. Each individual who serves as a member of a brigade does so voluntarily. However, the ultimate selection and assignment of a brigade member is made by the Area Emergency Supervisor and Fire Protection Department. Brigade members provide a pool of manpower who are responsible for implementing the emergency plans for their particular area or facility and certain outlying areas in emergency situations. This implementation may take the form of independent action or be part of a team response under the direction of the Area Emergency Supervisor and/or the Fire Captain at the scene.

Brigade members participate in emergency response training both within the area of assignment and from Laboratory-wide emergency response groups, i.e., Fire Protection Department, Plant Services, Industrial Hygiene and Radiation Safety. Through such training, brigade members and Laboratory-wide emergency response personnel become familiar with the equipment, areas and problems peculiar to both groups and are, therefore, more aware of the capabilities and limitations of both groups.

Monitors

In many of the areas, primarily the larger buildings which are composed of many wings or specific

areas under one roof, certain individuals are designated as monitors. The primary responsibility of
the individual monitor is to aid in emergencies which
require evacuation of their building or a particular
portion of the building to which they are assigned.
The monitor is the individual who makes certain that
all personnel in the affected area are aware of the
emergency and that evacuation when necessary is
complete. In addition, as part of the emergency
force, the monitor works closely with the Area
Emergency Supervisor and the occupants of his area
in evaluating the hazard potential of operations.

GROUP ALERTING SYSTEM

The Group Alerting System provides simultaneous telephonic contact between the individual reporting the emergency and all emergency response units.
This is the means by which emergency response personnel are initially and directly notified of an emergency. It is also the means used to terminate emergency operations.[3]
The Group Alerting System provides the flexibility
and efficiency demanded of a communication system
in meeting the needs of an emergency plan. Flexibility
and efficiency are maintained through the centralized
control of telephone and radio communications as well
as site-wide public address system.

Notification of an Emergency

The "DIAL 13 Procedure" was defined earlier as
the mechanism by which any individual can report

what he may consider to be an emergency. What
actually happens when the number "13" is dialed?
Upon receipt of a DIAL 13 at the central switchboard,
see Fig. 2, the Emergency Operator*[3] activates the
Group Alerting System and the emergency recorder.
Activation of this system simultaneously connects via
telephone the emergency response groups allowing
them to monitor the initial report of the emergency.
Emergency response groups are connected as indicated
in Fig. 3.

Incoming DIAL 13 calls to telephones on the Group
Alerting System are distinguishable from routine incoming calls in that the designated telephones ring
continuously until answered. In cases where telephones
on this system are in use at the time the Group Alerting System is activated, an overriding tone signal is
imposed thus alerting the users of the incoming emergency call. The Emergency Operator maintains the
capability to break into the conversation and advise
the users of the existence of an emergency situation
in cases where the overriding tone signal does not
obtain the necessary response. Assurance that all
emergency response units have received the DIAL 13
call is confirmed by the Emergency Operator.

The individual who dialed "13" is quiestioned by
the Fire Alarm Office Operator. A prepared list of

---

*Emergency Operator is the telephone switchboard
operator at the first position of the Laboratory's central switchboard. The Emergency Operator is responsible for the receipt and relay of emergency information. Notification of emergencies are normally
received by telephone; however, they may be received
by radio, alarm system, or messenger.

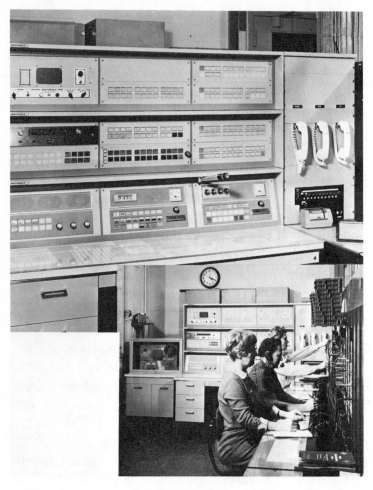

Fig. 2.   Emergency Control Center Console
and Switchboard

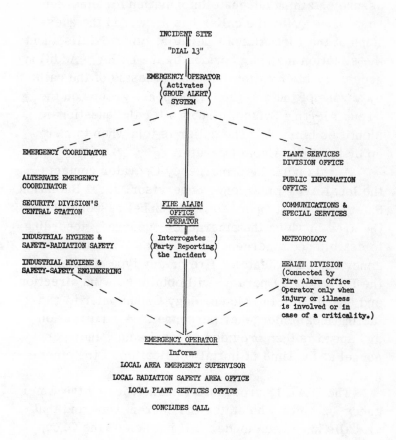

Fig. 3.   The ANL Group Alerting System.

questions is used by the Fire Alarm Operator to
assure obtaining adequate information for emergency
response. After the caller has answered the questions of the Fire Alarm Operator, other details about
the situation may be provided by the caller. Additional
necessary information may be requested of the caller
by anyone of the emergency response groups on the
Group Alerting System circuit after the questioner
identifies himself. The caller is told when to hang
up by the Fire Alarm Operator.

At this point the Emergency Operator contacts
the local Area Emergency Supervisor, local Radiation
Safety and Plant Operations personnel responsible for
the area in which the emergency occurred, according
to established emergency call lists. When the emergency report indicates a fire or any type of release,
the Emergency Operator will obtain the wind direction
and speed from the Meteorology Group prior to contacting local emergency personnel. Wind direction
and speed is then provided to local emergency personnel at the time of initial notification of the emergency.

The DIAL 13 procedure is concluded by the Emergency Operator who states the current time and that
all calls have been made. All parties on the Group
Alerting System hang up at this point.

Conclusion of an Emergency

The DIAL 13 procedure is used by the pertinent
Area Emergency Supervisor after he has determined
the emergency condition to be concluded, i.e., emergency operations are no longer required. Upon dialing "13", the Area Emergency Supervisor announces

the ALL CLEAR, and the Group Alerting System
carries this message to all parties previously
alerted.[3] The Emergency Operator upon receipt of
the ALL CLEAR from the Area Emergency Supervisor
utilizes the Laboratory emergency radio frequency to
inform emergency units the emergency condition has
ended.

Off-Shift Hours Operation

The Group Alerting System is modified during the
other than regular shift hours to meet the needs of
this period. Upon receipt of a DIAL 13 call during
the off-shift hours, the Emergency Operator activates
the Group Alerting System which connects only the
following emergency groups:[3] Fire Alarm Office
Operator, Security's Central Station, Health Division
and Meteorology. The caller is interrogated by the
Fire Alarm Operator as during normal working hours.
The Emergency Operator activates a five-second tone
signal which sounds inside and outside of all buildings
on the site-wide public address system and on the
emergency frequency of the radio system. The five-
second tone signal is utilized to inform the Radiation
Safety personnel and the Plant Services foreman that
a DIAL 13 call has been received and they are required to call the Emergency Operator who relays to
them the information provided by the caller. The
Emergency Operator makes separate calls to those
individuals who fail to respond to the site-wide five-
second tone signal and to the area maintenance man.
As pointed out in responsibilities of the Security
Lieutenant, he acts as the Emergency Coordinator and/
or Area Emergency Supervisor for all off-shift

emergencies. Therefore, the Security Lieutenant
initiates a DIAL 13 to report an ALL CLEAR at the
conclusion of the emergency conditions.

Indoctrination in the Reporting of Emergencies

Several means are employed to continuously provide instructional information regarding the DIAL 13
procedure to all employees and users of Laboratory
telephones.

Each telephone at the site has a decal affixed to
it upon installation. The decal highlights the number
"13" and how it should be dialed in any emergency.
It also bears the location of the telephone (building
and room number). [4] This decal has proved to be of
valuable assistance on many occasions when the stress
of the emergency conditions or lack of familiarity of
the particular area causes an uncertainty on the part
of the individual making the initial report of an incident.

Emergency instructions describing the standardized warning signals used throughout the site, special
signals, evacuation signals, Group Alerting System
and types of typical incidents, appears on the cover of
all Laboratory telephone directories.

A movie describing the DIAL 13 procedure has
been prepared by the Information Services Department. This movie is available to all employees and
is normally shown at certain scheduled safety meetings. It may also be screened by means of an 8 mm
continuous loop projector, a self-contained screening system which provides ready access to all employees. The DIAL 13 movie is utilized with the continuous loop projector at various times throughout the

year in the entrance lobbies of major buildings and
on-site cafeterias.

Major Emergency Procedure

The classification of an emergency situation as
a major emergency is the responsibility of the Area
Emergency Supervisor. Upon being advised that a
major emergency is in progress, the Emergency
Operator suspends normal activities and maintains a
constant alert as to the location of emergency personnel and the progress of emergency activities.
Arrangements have been made for a direct link between off-site line[2] and the telephone at the location
of the Emergency Coordinator in case the central
switchboard facility must be evacuated. Evacuation
would in no way disrupt usual dial service for outgoing calls by emergency units.

PREPLANNED ACTIONS

Up to this point the components of the basic plan:
Emergency Force Structure, Positions, Responsibilities and the Group Alerting System have been discussed. However, preplanned actions are essential
to any adequate emergency plan. Therefore, let us
consider one of the preplanned actions and its integration into the basic plan.

The Criticality Alarm System

Criticality is a special hazard which must be
considered in most nuclear facilities. So now let us
consider the Criticality Alarm System[5] as part of the
emergency plan.

Criticality detection devices and their associated control consoles, see Fig. 4, have been installed in twelve areas or facilities on site. Each criticality detection unit has one or more sensing devices and a sufficient number of alarm horns to provide adequate audible signal to the affected surrounding areas. The criticality alarm system has been designed so that many possible failures will result only in the activation of a buzzer at the control panel rather than in the activation of an evacuation alarm. The control panels and/or trouble buzzers are normally located in the local Radiation Safety Office and are under Radiation Safety control. However, the following situations will cause the alarm to sound: criticality producing neutron and gamma radiation; neutron or gamma radiation from other sources; severing of a detector cable; and, error in the manipulation of the control unit.

Power for the system is supplied by continually charged batteries and will continue to operate for four hours following total plant power failure. It may be repaired, tested and calibrated without interruption of service and has a response time of less than 1/2 second. The criticality alarm signals the Emergency Operator switchboard simultaneously with the sounding of the alarm in the building or facility in which the criticality was detected.

Indoctrination of Personnel in
Areas Served by Criticality Alarms

The primary purpose of the criticality alarm system is to provide a distinct audible warning to the occupants of any particular facility in the event a condition of criticality occurs. This system will

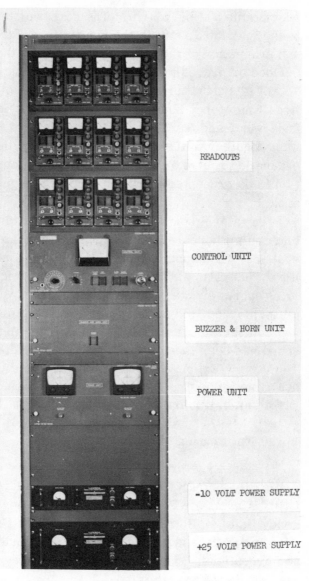

Figure 4.
Criticality detection control console.

provide the audible alarm. The next two steps are up
to the individual, that is the recognition of the alarm
and evacuation of the facility according to the prescribed or predesignated routes. The designation of
approved evacuation routes is the responsibility of the
Area Emergency Supervisor. The Area Emergency
Supervisor and the assigned Health Physicist should
work together in the evaluation and determination of
evacuation routes and developing instructional information to be presented to all individuals assigned to their
area.

The alarm sound consists of a loud intermittent
blast on all horns connected to the particular building
system. The sound quality of the alarm horn is similar to that of an air horn used by large vehicles and/
or at sports events. To facilitate the instruction of
all employees, old and new alike, Laboratory visitors
and contractor personnel, the criticality alarm horn
sound has been taped and can be heard by dialing
Laboratory Extension 4761. A taped message is also
available for instructional purposes in each area which
has a criticality alarm system.

Initial Notification of a Criticality Incident

Emergency forces are initially notified of a
criticality as outlined in a detailed procedure: Criticality Alarms—A Procedure for Notification of Emergency Units. [5] However, in summary: the Group
Alerting System is utilized as described prior with
two exceptions: (1) notification is usually by alarm at
the emergency switchboard. Therefore, the Emergency Operator reports: the alarm and wind speed and
direction to the parties on the Group Alerting System

directly; (2) Communications and Special Services
Division personnel monitor all emergency calls on the
Group Alerting System. Therefore, upon notification
of a criticality alarm, Communications and Special
Services personnel make an announcement via both
assigned radio frequencies, informing all service
vehicles and on-site taxis of the alarm and advises
them to stay clear of the area. Notification of a
criticality during off-shift hours follows the pattern
of the off-shift DIAL 13 procedure.

Actions and Responsibilities
of Emergency Response Units[5]

Each of the groups required to respond to a criticality alarm develops appropriate detailed plans within their organization to meet their responsibilities.
A criticality incident requires a quick initial response
from the emergency forces. General preplanned
actions and responsibilities of certain response units
are described below:
The Area Emergency Supervisor provides emergency units with necessary instructions; to actively
direct emergency operations at the scene during the
regular shift hours. He is responsible for the
designation of evacuation routes for the buildings or
facilities in his area.
The Area Emergency Supervisor or his alternate
is normally notified of a criticality incident in his
building or facility by the sounding of the building
criticality alarm horn during the regular shift. If the
physical characteristics of the normal location of the
Area Emergency Supervisor and his alternate are such
that there is the possibility either one or both might

not be able to hear the alarm horns, the responsibility for contacting Communications and Special Services, and arranging for appropriate alarms, buzzer, etc. lies with the Area Emergency Supervisor.

Radiation Safety personnel measure and evaluate radiation fields, contamination, advise on exposure matters in order to minimize radiation exposure and contamination, and to assist the Area Emergency Supervisor in evaluation and designation of evacuation routes.

Fire Protection Department personnel aid in rescue operations and the control of associated fires, should they exist. They provide at the scene a source of equipment, for example: ladders, lights, supplied air breathing apparatus, stokes stretcher, and other rescue type items and personnel trained in their use.

Security Division personnel establish appropriate traffic control measures in order to expedite evacuation and prevent the access of other than emergency personnel to the incident areas. They provide assistance in collection of information and control of personnel evacuated at the evacuation assembly point.

The Security Lieutenant provides notification of off-shift criticality incidents to appropriate emergency force and management representatives according to a prearranged list at his earliest convenience. If the investigation of the criticality alarm determines the incident to have been a false alarm or some other minor problem, the Security Lieutenant provides notification as appropriate concerning the incident, based on his evaluation at that time.

Meteorology personnel provide pertinent information on present and immediately forecasted weather conditions and advise on their expected effects on the incident situation.

Health Division personnel arrange and provide for the administration of appropriate medical treatment and arrange patient transportation.

Special Materials and Services Division personnel provide pertinent information regarding the location, amounts, physical nature and storage conditions of fissionable materials to the emergency response personnel.

OTHER PREPLANNED ACTIVITIES

Preplanning activities in preparation for emergencies must also fit the descriptive terms of the overall plan: flexibility and efficiency.   A few examples of preplanning activities of certain emergency response groups are described in the following paragraphs.

Checklists

One of the major contributing causes to most emergency situations is the lack of thoroughness on the part of an individual, reaction, mechanical or electronic control or other equipment. Similarly a lack of thoroughness on the part of individuals responsible for handling an emergency can compound an already serious situation.   Certain emergency force groups have prepared checklists which they use as a guide in handling their particular aspects of an emergency situation. One such checklist appears as Appendix I. [6] Users of checklists should be advised that such lists are to be used as guides and/or reminders but should not replace common sense.

Emergency Cabinets

Another approach to handling emergencies is by utilization of emergency cabinets. One-hundred-and-thirteen (113) emergency cabinets have been located within buildings throughout the site, at or near operational areas. The cabinets provide tools and protective equipment which can be utilized in rescue of trapped or injured personnel or shutting down equipment and facilities.

The cabinets are mounted on casters to allow movement to an area of easy accessibility in emergency situations. The contents of the cabinets are shown in Fig. 5. Certain items in the cabinets require maintenance and routine testing, e.g., batteries, rope, respirator canisters, supplied breathing air apparatus, and high voltage gloves. These tests and other routine inspections are carried out by Radiation Safety personnel. Radiation Safety personnel, Area Emergency Supervisors and pertinent divisional representatives assist in the determination of need, location, stocking of these cabinets. Certain Laboratory-wide emergency response organizations provide training sessions on the use of items contained in the cabinets.

Building Emergency Packets[7]

In a large research facility, experimental apparatus, levels of materials and equipment locations are constantly changing. It is difficult for a limited number of site-wide emergency response personnel to maintain detailed knowledge of the physical layout and significant modifications of all areas which could be considered potentially hazardous. In an effort to overcome this problem and to provide

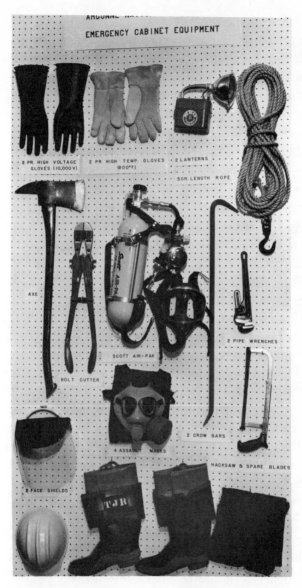

Fig. 5.   A Display of the Contents of Emergency Cabinets.

emergency rescue and recovery personnel with current detailed information, the Building Emergency
Packets were developed. Each building which houses
a potentially hazardous operation(s) has an emergency
packet prepared and maintained for use by emergency
response groups. A Building Emergency Packet contains: engineering drawings of each floor and/or level
of the building or facility; "as built" photographs of
potentially hazardous operations as seen from the en-
trances with appropriate legend information; and a
listing of all buildings throughout the site which is
considered to house a potential major accident. The
primary and alternate (nearby buildings), Decontamination and/or Control Centers are listed along side each
potential major accident building.

On each engineering drawing certain permanent
or semipermanent items used in the evaluation and
control of emergencies have been indicated by a
standardized marking system. Items so indicated are:
nuclear accident dosimeters; constant air samplers
other than CAM-5's; permanent film badge and dosimeter racks; rover dosimeter racks, continuous air
monitors CAM-5's; Savannah River dosimeters; and
emergency cabinets.

The development of a system of emergency
packets is no small chore. However, the system is
no more than an uninteresting record of "the way
things used to be" unless each packet reflects the
current conditions. Radiation Safety personnel review the potentially hazardous areas on a monthly
basis. Photographs are made and updated as needed
according to general guidelines. The entire packet
of each building is totally reviewed quarterly.

Six identical emergency packets are maintained
for each building requiring a packet. One copy of
each building emergency packet is maintained by
Radiation Safety personnel in the following locations:
Communications and Special Services (Emergency
Control Center); Radiation Safety Section Supervisor's
Office; Fire Protection Department Alarm Office;
Radiation Safety Area Office of the Pertinent Area;
Area Emergency Supervisor's Office or Building
Emergency Control Center of the Pertinent Building;
and Radiation Safety Office of a Specified Building.

It can be argued that such a system is difficult to
maintain and costly. The cost of photographs used in
establishing the system (22 Building Emergency
Packets) is insignificant when compared to their value
in time of need. As for maintenance, the schedule for
review serves as the primary reminder to those
responsible to be continually vigilant of potential
incident areas. A close review of the description of
many previous incidents has often indicated the lack
of and need for detailed knowledge of the facility and
equipment location. The Building Emergency Packets
serve this purpose. These packets have proved to be
a valuable source of information in controlling minor
emergencies.

Radiological Assistance Team[8]

In cooperation with the Chicago Operations Office
of the Atomic Energy Commission, Argonne supplies
a Radiological Assistance Team as part of the Interagency Radiological Assistance Plan. The Team is
composed of twelve members of the Industrial Hygiene
and Safety Division. The capability of this emergency

response unit was primarily designed to provide self-contained emergency radiological assistance at the scene of off-site emergencies involving radiation. This primary purpose (off-site assistance) has been utilized on fifty occasions since the Team was organized in 1957. The capabilities, personnel and equipment of this organization are available for on-site assistance in emergency situations at the request and under direct control of the Radiation Safety Supervisor. An emergency equipped vehicle, see Fig. 6, set aside for the sole use of the Team provides a mobile unit manned by personnel trained and experienced in handling emergencies who are capable of obtaining meaningful results from analysis made under field type operating conditions. The Team equipment also includes: 3.5 kW of AC power, two radio frequency links with emergency forces, a public address system and a limited emergency lighting capability.

Identification of Emergency Response Personnel

Many specific positions within the emergency force structure have been described along with their general and specific duties. Identification of specific individuals at the site of an emergency becomes difficult as all individuals who respond are not attired in a manner which denotes differentiation or designation of their particular responsibility. In many instances respiratory protective devices and other protective equipment obscure the faces of responding individuals. Therefore, arm bands, which can conveniently fit in a shirt pocket, have been prepared and provided those individuals who are required to respond to emergencies.

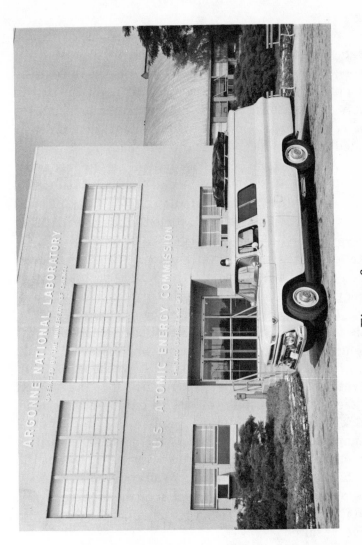

Figure 6.

The emergency vehicle which is equipped and reserved for the use of the Interagency Radiological Assistance Team.

SUMMARY

Argonne's emergency plan is directed toward the protection of personnel and the minimization of property damage. It can be seen from the description of the basic plan, its controlling positions and their responsibilities that the overall plan provides the necessary framework for the integration of detailed plans of the individual emergency response units. A means of initiating and halting emergency activities was detailed in the description of the Group Alerting System. One example of integration of such plans is presented in the description of the criticality alarm system and the listing of responsibilities of particular response groups. Other examples of preplanned aids were described, i.e., checklists, emergency cabinets and building emergency packets.

The aspects of the emergency plan described in this paper comprise only a small part of the entire plan. Many valuable innovations and expanded capabilities have resulted from the efforts expended in the development of the emergency plan. It is the opinion of the author that the present day emergency forces working together within the framework of the emergency plan successfully handle incidents and situations which are casually considered routine. However, if such incidents and situations had occurred prior to the present state of development of the emergency plan, it is conceivable that major emergencies could have resulted.

ACKNOWLEDGMENTS

The author wishes to acknowledge the assistance of J. R. Novak, V. H. Munnecke, J. R. Sanecki, W. H. Smith and R. Omiecinski who made valuable comments, Majorie Bobysud who assisted in the preparation of the paper and the many unnamed employees who have over the years participated in the development of the Laboratory's Emergency Plan.

APPENDIX I

RADIATION SAFETY CONTROL CENTER PROCEDURE CHECK

The procedures listed herein should be considered as a guide or aid in handling incident situations. The order of consideration of the individual items listed should be determined to suit the particular incident.

Personnel

1. Are all personnel involved at incident site accounted for?

2. Have personnel been surveyed?

    a) Are personnel segregated as to contamination and/or induced activity levels?

    b) Injuries noted?

    c) Has decontamination been attempted and results noted?

    d) Were personnel monitoring devices collected?

    e) Have all pertinent data pertaining to personnel been remanded to Health Division?

3.   Have personnel downwind of the incident been notified?

4.   Have the proper bioassay procedures been initiated?

    a) Samples from persons involved?

    b) Samples from persons injured with contamination or suspect contamination material?

    c) Persons downwind?

    d) Persons subsequently involved?

    e) Have sample kits been distributed?

    f) Have sample kits been returned?

    g) Have data been submitted to bioassay?

    h) Have results been received?

    i) Have results been reported to pertinent authority?

5.   Have measures been instituted to control ingress and egress of personnel into hazard area?

    a) Guards been notified?

    b) Communications and Special Services n notified?

    c) Barriers erected?

6. Have measures been instituted to protect personnel on re-entry?

    a) Protective clothing and shoe covers.

    b) Respiratory equipment.

    c) Knowledge of radiation hazard.

    d) Knowledge of other hazards.

Evaluation

1. Have surveys been made outside of the control area?

    a) Radiological Assistance Team utilized?

    b) Air samples taken downwind?

    c) Peripheral surveys made?

    d) Surveys made of vehicles and/or equipment used in incident?

    e) Have "continuous operation" instruments been checked for data?

    f) Personnel monitor device results been recorded?

2. Have surveys been made of the incident area?

    a) Contamination levels?

    b) Background levels?

    c) Air samples taken and recorded?

    d) Accident dosimeters retrieved?

3. Have contacts been initiated with personnel familiar with the incident facility?

    a) Personnel involved, if possible?

    b) Plant Services for that area?

    c) Plant Engineering?

    d) Others?

Instrumentation and Equipment

1. Has sufficient instrumentation been acquired?

    a) Portable.

    b) Alternating current counters.

    c) Analyzers.

    d) Air samplers (Particulate and Gas).

    e) Portable alternating current generators (when needed).

2. Is an instrument repairman on hand for limited repair work?

Protective Apparel

Has sufficient apparel been procured?

    a) Coveralls.

    b) Underclothing.

    c) Shoe covers.

    d) Gloves.

Respiratory Devices

Is there a supply of proper respirators to meet the need?

    a) Scott Air Paks.

    b) Supplied-air suits.

    c) Assault Masks and canisters.

    d) Dust respirators.

    e) Other.

Control

1.   Have measures been instituted to contain the incident?

    a) Fire extinguishers.

    b) Ventilation shutdown (when needed).

    c) Cause area isolated.

    d) Utilities secured.

    e) Hazard area isolated.

    f) Shoe cover change areas and survey points set up.

2.   Have measures been taken to insure against recurrence of incident?

    a) Discussion with personnel familiar with incident apparatus.

    b) Assistance in developing methods of neutralization of incident apparatus.

Transportation

Are there sufficient vehicles on hand?

a) General transportation.

b) Survey vehicles.

c) Decontamination vehicles (bulldozers, road graders, tankers, etc.).

d) Other.

Communications

Have communications been established?

a) Telephone.

b) Mobile radio.

c) Portable radio.

d) Laboratory radio.

Plant and Facilities (Immediate)

Have measures been taken to reduce the loss or damage to plant equipment?

a) Secure utilities.

b) Neutralize destructive conditions (fires, acids, water, etc.).

Plant and Facilities (Restoration)

Have measures been taken to restore facilities?

a) Assist in developing techniques with proper authorities.

b) Consult with Reclamation Services (decontamination).

Security

Have proper measures been taken to safeguard security items and/or areas?

Reporting

Is a running log of events and data being complied?

a) Survey of personnel.

b) Personnel exposures.

c) Survey of periphery.

d) Survey immediate area.

e) Bioassay results.

f) Manpower used.

g) Instrumentation and equipment used.

h) Progress of control

i) Control measures taken.

Have the Radiation Safety activities been reported to proper authority?

a) Laboratory Director or authorized representative.

b) Technical Services Manager.

c) Laboratory Control Center.

d) Other.

REFERENCES

1. "What is Argonne National Laboratory",
    Argonne, Illinois, (May 1968).

2. "Emergency Handbook ANL", unpublished,
    Argonne, Illinois, July 1966.

3. V. H. Munnecke, "Group Alerting System",
    Announcement to All Employees, Argonne
    National Laboratory, Argonne Illinois,
    October 25. 1967.

4. J. T. Sanecki and D. L. Matson, Argonne y,
    National Laboratory, Private Communica-
    tion, Argonne, Illinois, Dec. 1968.

5. "Criticality Alarms--A Procedure for Noti-
    fication of Emergency Units", Unpublished
    Procedure, Argonne National Laboratory,
    Argonne, Illinois, (Revised), October, 1968.

6. W. H. Smith, N. C. Dyer, and G. T. Lonergan,
    Unpublished Internal Report, Argonne National
    Laboratory, May 1962, incorporated as an
    Appendix in Radiation Accident and Emergencies
    in Medicine, Research and Industry, edited by
    Lanzl, L. H., Pingel, J. H., and Rust, J. H.,
    Charles C. Thomas publisher, Springfield,
    Illinois, 1965.

7. F. L. Bordell, A. G. Januska, S. R. Lasuk, C. D. Hampleman, T. M. Tongue and L. H. Sprouse, Unpublished Internal Committee Reports (1961-66), Argonne National Laboratory, Argonne, Illinois.

8. G. T. Lonergan and W. H. Smith, Radiological Assistance Team, ANL-6786, October, 1963.

ROLE OF THE HEALTH PHYSICIST IN A NUCLEAR ATTACK

Harold W. Gaut
Radiological Defense Officer
DOA/OSA, OCD Region Two
Olney, Maryland

I should like to describe for your consideration a maximum credible incident. Mixed fission products and some unfissioned fuel material, fused to a generally insoluble particulate carrier, have been deposited in varying concentrations ranging up to one hundred gamma curies per square meter over an area of almost 3 million square miles. The principal hazard from this material is a series of gamma emitters having an average energy of approximately 1 MeV and a probable exponential decay rate of approximately $t^{-1.2}$ where t is in units of time from 1 hour to several weeks after the incident. It should be noted that this decay rate is variable due to the possible presence of certain neutron activated materials, fractionation and distribution of particle sizes during production of the contaminant and weather conditions in the area of interest. Operational resources may or may not be readily available and the population at risk may only be adequately protected for a limited period. Failure to effectively react, to evaluate, overcome, control and correct the situation could seriously damage the population and resources of the United States.

Such is the situation in which we might find ourselves in the event of a nuclear attack involving in excess of 100 or so megaton size weapons. While I am not going to debate, at this point, the probability of such an attack, nor the means of its implementation, its credibility is an accepted fact. The fact that it is credible means it must be planned for and the gravity of the resulting situation indicates the pressing need for high quality technical support.

Such a disaster would lean heavily on a major countermeasure system of Civil Defense, namely Radiological Defense. Radiological Defense or RADEF is defined as "The Organized Effort through Detection, Warning, and Preventive and Remedial Measures to Minimize the Effect of Nuclear Radiation on People and Resources." Obviously, the effectiveness of RADEF as a countermeasure will be directly proportional to the competence, experience, ingenuity and proficiency displayed by the individuals involved.

The origins of health physics and RADEF are much alike. Health physics was born with the advent of the first sustained chain reaction under the stands of Stagg Field in 1942. Radiological Defense could probably be said to have been conceived on the flats of the New Mexico Desert in 1945, or, if not then, certainly in 1954 in the Pacific as a result of tests with high yield nuclear weapons and extensive fallout.

The problem in either case is a common one, the threat of biological damage to people and their environment from uncontrolled radiation.

The objectives of health physics and Radiological Defense are also basically the same, varying only in the priority of the emphasis. In peace-time we seek two NCRP objectives: fewest persons exposed and least exposure to them. In a nuclear war our objectives would be first, fewest deaths; second, fewest casualities; third, minimum genetic injury; and last, minimum late somatic effects. Extrapolation of peace-time objectives brings them right in line with those of Civil Defense. Finally, the time phasing of the operations in health physics and RADEF are very similar in that each has an emergency phase, in which the objective is basically to preserve all useable resources; an operational recovery phase, in which the objective is to minimize exposure while reestablishing essential functions; and a final recovery phase in which we try to return to normal operations. As most operational health physicists are painfully aware, the ability to react in all of these phases will be predicated upon one major phase which I have not yet mentioned. That phase is one which precedes all other actions and concerns itself with planning.

PLANNING

Accepting the fact that the early post attack environment is part and parcel of a massive radiological incident, we must then analyze what planning objectives are required in order to cope with it effectively.

Initially, we must have a source of information
on the extent of the problem. To accomplish this we
must establish a basic monitoring system and administrative channels for prompt reporting of dose and
dose rate information. We must also have convenient
and reliable sources of meteorological data, especially winds aloft.

Without the capability for rapid assimilation and
utilization of such data at the point of receipt, however, the effectiveness of any operation is still pre-
carious at best. Therefore, trained technical teams
must be assembled in emergency operating centers to
make optimum use of available data.

In order to remain abreast of the situation all
data will have to be updated periodically. To this
end we must be sure that we do not have a one-shot
reporting system but rather one which is capable of
sustained operation without inflicting grave biological
damage on the individuals manning it. Directly involved here then is the geographical and sheltered
placement of monitoring stations.

Even before we have first-hand knowledge of
actual conditions, we must make certain assumptions
upon which we can form contingency plans which in
turn will allow us to react faster as actual facts become known. After determining the possible contingencies that may present themselves, implementation plans for priority recovery measures must be
constructed.

For example, plans must be made for decontamination of vital facilities, protection of people, possible
relocation of people from weak shelters to where we
know that there are good shelters not yet filled to
capacity.

In any case, since we have a major area which must be cleaned up and reoccupied as soon as possible, the effective marshalling of exposure control will be vital to the survival of the teams, as well as timely accomplishment of the mission. To this end we must not think in terms of actual man-hours of work but rather effective man-roentgens of exposure, including the background dose received by off duty operating personnel.

OPERATIONS

In the operational phase of a nuclear attack the RADEF Officer will have prime responsibility for the deployment and coordination of monitoring teams. The quality of these teams will be a function of the training which he has been able to ensure that they have. The RADEF Officer will be relied upon by the Emergency head of Government, through his delegated representatives, the Civil Defense Director, to prognosticate the radiological situation which will exist at certain periods of time in the future. These prognostications will have to be made based on his knowledge of the contaminant, wheather patterns, and the capability to field decontamination and recovery teams. Based on his prognosis he will have to review formulated plans of action and recommend among them, with accompanying explanations of the resulting radiological effects of each, to the Civil Defense Director. This last action will be expedited in direct proportion to the quality of the contingency plans which were made up pre-attack. In every case the Director will need enough information to effectively weigh the

hazard and urgency of a given action or mission.
Concurrently with the above activity the RADEF
Officer will be continuously required to present to the
Civil Defense Director, in a useable and understand-
able form, data which he has assimilated from his
monitoring teams. In this case then we are faced
with a situation where the RADEF Officer must not
only be able to communicate with his technical counterpart but also with nontechnical supervisory staff who
are charged with making decisions.

The capabilities of RADEF are principally oriented
towards the detection of the high range gamma emitter in the early post attack period. To this end our
detection capabilities are basically dependent on
geiger counters, high range ion chambers, and beta-
gamma dosimeters. We are not overly concerned
with the problem of prompt neutrons nor of alpha and
soft beta emitting materials in the fallout. At such
time, post attack, as the latter do become the principle hazard, technical responsibilities will gradually
revert to a number of other specialized agencies until
final recovery is accomplished.

It should be noted, in passing, that because of the
potential alpha and soft beta contaminant, a RADEF
organization should not inject itself, alone, into
peacetime nuclear accidents but should defer to
specialized teams.

TRAINING

Any organization requires some specialized
training for its various personnel. In RADEF we have
Radiological Defense Officers; Assistant RADEF

Officers, normally recruited from qualified individuals who serve as monitor instructors pre-attack; monitors or meter readers; emergency operations staff comprized of plotters and analysts; and emergency decontamination teams. All of these personnel have some specialized courses which they may attend. To the extent that they will assist in solidifying concepts of radiological defense and war oriented disasters, any of the courses would be useful to the health physicist.

There is also the aspect of public information, or the training of the populace in adapting their attitudes towards a disaster situation. This is no stranger to the health physicist since the science fiction effects of radiation have always been a major block in his quest to educate the public to the realistic hazards of radiation. If the bent of the health physicist is towards the instructional, he can be of great value by assisting in or conducting training courses for his community or industrial complex. He can also prepare material for inclusion in the professional development, and ABHP exam preparation courses presented by most local chapters.

Finally, after operational assignments are made and training is completed, systems must be exercised. In constructing and implementing these exercises the health physicist will have ample practice in all of the planning and operational aspects discussed earlier.

While I have had to move rather quickly, an expanded and more detailed presentation of all planning and operations aspects of RADEF is given in the Appendices to Part E, Chapter 5 of the Federal Civil Defense Guide, available from State and Regional Civil Defense Offices.

ORGANIZATION

At this point I feel we must firmly establish that
Civil Defense is merely a formal designation for
Government in an emergency. In peacetime a small
staff is concerned with this responsibility, with its
principal emphasis being on the development of a
fallout shelter program and community shelter
planning. It works with and assists other government
agencies, in developing their plans and, training their
personnel for emergency operations. In an emergency
the same staff becomes the coordinating agency for
all the resources that exist day-to-day, such as fire
and police departments, welfare organizations and
so on, while the State Civil Defense Director becomes,
by way of example, the Chief of Staff to the Governor.
      Necessary emergency specialities can be found
in Federal, State, and Local Governments as part of
their normal operating groups with one exception.
This exception is radiological defense. At the State
and Federal levels, a basis for this capability can be
found in agencies such as the AEC, Public Health
Service, and State Health Departments. However,
with the exception of major metropolitan areas it does
not normally exist at the local level. It is vital that
this void be filled at local level since this is where
the success or failure of our efforts will be reward-
ingly or tragically demonstrated. We must bear in
mind that without a vigorous RADEF capability, any
recovery operations, because of the unique threat of
fallout, will be seriously hampered. The Federal
Office of Civil Defense, a part of the Office of the
Secretary of the Army, provides guidance and assistance, financial and otherwise, to the States and their

political subdivisions in developing capability for
emergency operations, in accordance with Public Law
920, 81st Congress.

SUMMARY

Based on the foregoing discussion I think that the
following postulate can be stated: Radiological Defense
and health physics are the same vehicle powered by
the same technical engine being driven towards the
same goal of radiation protection. The only difference
is a shifting of gears on the part of the health physicist. A corollary to this then would be that, as more
health physicists become gear shifters they will discover in radiological defense many challenging new
areas for investigation and application in direct proportion to their resourcefulness and experience.

Civil Defense is merely an organized effort of
the civilian population to react intelligently and re-
cover in the event of a major debilitating incident
brought on by an external cause. RADEF is a major
countermeasure system of that effort. The human
resources that radiological defense has available to
it are to be found in industry, government, or the
educational system. With such a broad choice, there
is a tendancy to "let George do it." Assume that the
health physicist does not react to the need. Then who
does speak for radiation protection in a nuclear
attack?

In August of 1966 an Ad Hoc committee on civil
defense reported to the Board of Directors of our
society. I would like to share certain portions of
their report with you. It commences with the

statement that "in many ways the mission of the Health
Physics Society and Civil Defense Organizations are
complementary. The one is devoted to ensuring that
useful procedures involving radiation are carried out
with a minimum of radiation exposure. The other is
charged with planning so that radiation injury and
death shall be minimized in the event of a major peace-
time disaster or hostile military action." The great
difference in magnitude between the two situations is
emphasized and the caution is put forth that those who
associate with civil defense must be those who can
adapt to the uniqueness of the situation. The report
goes on to state, in its suggested guidelines, that
"Many members of the Health Physics Society have
technical competencies and operational experiences
that could be of considerable help to Civil Defense
organizations." Of special interest here is your own
local Civil Defense group since it will probably have
the strongest influence on the environment in which
your day-to-day operation may ultimately have to
function.

In closing let me say that as health physicists,
our coin has two sides. The Civil Defense can receive
many benefits from our technical assistance since
radiation protection is our stock in trade. We on the
other hand can gain the benefits of a broadened spectrum of knowledge by participation in the special
problems generated during the development of a sound
radiological defense operation.

WEAPON EFFECTS TESTS—PLANNED EMERGENCIES*

Harold L. Rarrick
Sandia Laboratories
Albuquerque, New Mexico

INTRODUCTION

Radiation emergencies usually involve the following parameters:

1. A large source of radiation released to the environment.

2. Recovery of valuable property or information.

3. Unknown contamination, external radiation, and air concentration levels.

4. Necessary reentry of personnel into the area.

5. High levels of induced radioactivity in materials to be recovered.

---

*This work was supported by the United States Atomic Energy Commission.

These characteristic elements also define a weapon effects test. Since 1957 the Health Physics Division of Sandia Laboratories has participated in the recovery of experiments both for the Laboratories and for the Department of Defense. In these 12 years, a number of problems have obviously been encountered.

DISCUSSION

To illustrate selective problems and the solutions we have arrived at, I want to discuss three types of weapons effects tests.

The first type can be illustrated by the Small Boy event, a low-yield nuclear detonation on July 14, 1962 at NTS. The device was located slightly aboveground.[1] The Sandia Laboratories had a number of experiments located in bunkers at 150 and 250 feet from ground zero. Since the bunkers were within fireball radius, the entire area was covered with fused silica containing fission products. When recovery operations were started about one month after the event, radiation levels at the rear bunker were about 12 R/hr and at the forward bunker were up to 40 R/hr.

The first step was to remove the fused silica. We used a grader, a bulldozer, and a water truck to settle the dust. After the immediate areas around the bunkers were scraped, laborers knocked the slag off the bunkers. All these efforts reduced the radiation field to about one R/hr, which was entirely acceptable for recovery work.

Since the free air temperature was in excess of 130° F, we went to considerable effort to keep the area watered to avoid making people work in face masks.

The point to be made here is that with careful planning, adequate equipment and willingness to accept permissible radiation doses, people can rapidly decrease radiation-contaminated areas to acceptable levels for limited operations.

The second type of test can be illustrated by a research program jointly conducted by the AEC, DOD and the United Kingdom for the evaluation of accidental non-nuclear detonation of plutonium-bearing weapons (Operation Roller Coaster).[2] The program included four experimental detonations, three of which were on the Sandia Laboratories' Tonopah Test Range. One of our responsibilities was to restore the Test Range to its pre-test condition as a ballistics, rocket and parachute testing site. Where this was not possible, the job was to minimize the remaining personnel hazards and interferences with future range operations.

The detonations yielded molten plutonium metal that combined with device materials, earth, concrete and metal.

On one exposed detonation on top of the ground, radiological health hazards consisted of minor earth throw-out to 100 yards, and dust fallout up to ten miles.

Detonations two and three were bunker shots. The hazards were large volumes of earth, concrete and metal debris, scattered up to 2500 feet, with dust fall-out up to 7 miles. Extensive rains shortly after the detonation leached the bulk of the downwind fallout into the soil. The problems of low-level fallout and resuspension were, therefore, considerably diminished.

The debris in the vicinity of the ground zero areas and the fragments out to a range of 2500 feet were

collected and buried inside the ground zero areas.
The contaminated surface was scraped to a depth of
several inches. This soil was placed in the debris
hole, compacted and watered. The ground zero areas
were fenced outside the compacted areas and posted.
Large warning signs were placed on roads leading
into the area.

Although ground contamination of 10,000 cpm per
60 cm^2 still exists, the contamination is fixed on
larger particles of sand and dirt. No significant contamination has been found in other areas of the test
range nor on any vehicles used in the area.

I would like to discuss just briefly the third type
(tests in tunnels). The recovery of some experiments
involves returning up to 7000 feet into a mountain.
The possible hazards are:[3]

1. Radiation due to leaks or failure of the
    stemming.

2. Explosive and toxic gases resulting from the
    detonation.

3. Unexploded explosives associated with the
    test.

4. Tunnel damage generated by the shock wave.

To anticipate the problems, we use about 50
channels of remote radiation monitoring that is read
out up to 30 miles away.

We have a gas monitoring system throughout the
tunnel complex. Samples are analyzed with a gas
chromatograph located outside the tunnel. We also
maintain remote control over various options of
ventilation.

When it appears from studies that the tunnel is safe, we enter, using two-hour oxygen breathing apparatus. Constant communication is maintained with the reentry party by means of hard-wire lines.

All unsealed drifts in the tunnel are walked out and monitored, and any tunnel damage is repaired by the reentry teams. After this is accomplished, the lights are turned on and recovery of the experiments takes place.

As you can see, we have developed three different types of operations that would, if not planned before-hand, be regarded as emergencies. I believe that the techniques and experience gained in the weapon test program are applicable to the planning for emergency actions. I see particular relevance to standard mine rescue operations, for example.

REFERENCES

1. Effect of Nuclear Weapons, Revised edition, February, 1964.

2. William D. Burnett, Harold L. Rarrick, and George E. Tucker Jr., Health Physics Aspects of Operation Roller Coaster, Sandia Laboratories, SC-4973 (RR), January, 1964.

3. G. R. Wenz, and H. L. Rarrick, General Tunnel Reentry Procedures for Department of Defense and Sandia Laboratory Nuclear Tests, Sandia Laboratories, SC-M-68-227, April, 1968.

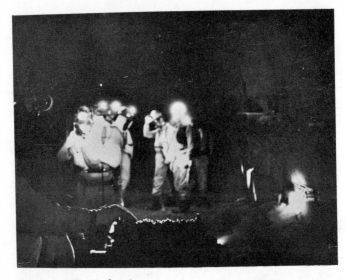

Fig. 1. Reentry Party in Tunnel.

RAMS, Wind Velocity and Direction, and Ventilation Flow Rate Chart Recorders

Fig. 2. RAMS, Wind Velocity and Direction, and Ventilation Flow Rate Chart Recorders.

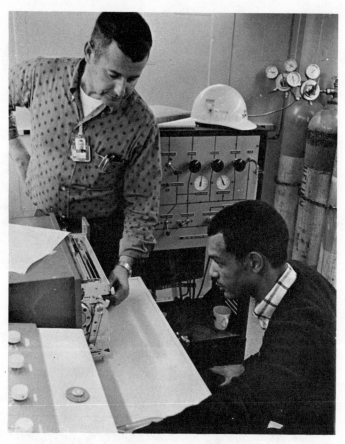

Fig. 3.   Gas Sampling System-Chromatograph
in Left Foreground.

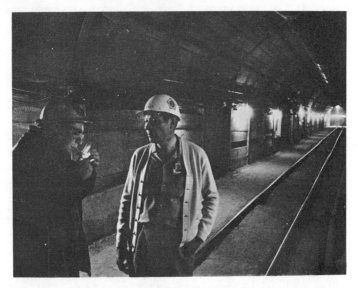

Fig. 4. Typical Tunnel Construction

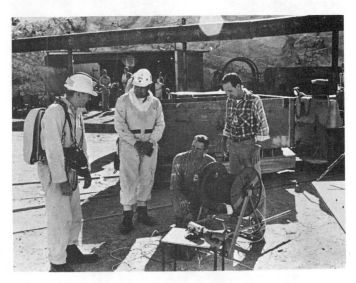

Fig. 5.   Portal Areas Draeger 2 Hour Oxygen
Breathing System on Left, Reel for Communication Cable in Foreground.

RADIOLOGICAL EMERGENCY EXPERIENCE IN AN INDUSTRIAL PLUTONIUM PLANT

Roger Caldwell, Thomas Potter and Edward Schnell
Nuclear Materials and Equipment Corporation
Apollo, Pennsylvania

".... Truth is discovered by way of experience"
—Roger Bacon

As long as man exists, there will be accidents. Even the most elaborate safety rules and regulations won't entirely prevent industrial accidents. There is always an element of the unforeseen, which will confound the best laid plans of man.

Manufacturers and users of radioactive materials are not exempt from industrial accidents. In fact, industrial type accidents in radioactive materials plants are often complicated by the radiation hazards. What would ordinarily be a trivial accident in a non-nuclear plant, may become a serious problem in a nuclear plant, because of an invisible amount of contamination.

NUMEC has had four serious accidents at its Plutonium Plant. Our facility, the world's first

commercial Plutonium Laboratory, is located near
Leechburg, Pennsylvania. We should mention that
the plant operated for five years before the first
accident occurred. We will describe each accident,
what our emergency response was and how we recovered from the accident. At the end of the article,
we will summarize what we have learned about preventing accidents, minimizing contamination complications and assuring good response to future emergencies.

1. DRY BOX EXPLOSION,
JANUARY 17, 1966

At 2:05 p.m. a glove box exploded, when a
technician struck a sparker inside the box to light a
propane torch. Apparently the torch leaked, after a
new cylinder was attached. The explosion blew out
the box gloves and knocked the technician to the floor.
Hot gases from the open glove ports singed the
operator's eye brows and produced minor first degree burns, but he had no other physical injury.

The technician spread contamination, when he
ran out of the room with box gloves still on his arms.
Alpha contamination ranged up to 100,000 c/m on the
technician's hair, face and chest. A nose smear,
taken before showering, measured 50,000 d/m. He
was decontaminated at the plutonium plant to less than
1000 c/m. The remaining skin contamination re-
sisted further decon efforts.

Fully protected emergency personnel entered the
contaminated room within minutes to put out fires
started in the affected glove box. They placed covers

on open ports, surveyed the area and sealed off the room. Alpha floor activity in the accident vicinity ranged up to 300,000 c/m/100 cm^2. Air Samples, running during the accident, indicated 10-20 minute concentrations up to 1.1 x 10^{-7} μCi/ml or the equivalent of 367 MPC-hours (considering ^{241}AmO$_2$ as the contaminant. At the time of the accident we assumed ^{239}PuO$_2$ and thought the exposure was more than 900 MPC-hours).

After attending to the exposed technician, our most immediate problem was identifying other potentially contaminated personnel. One hundred and fifty employees were present in the plant, and since contamination was spread through the plant, we were not sure who was exposed. Every one was monitored externally and shepherded into the plant cafeteria. Nasal smears, taken on all personnel, showed that only the involved technician had been seriously exposed.

Our Health Physics Laboratory became "buried" by the incident, because it was in the controlled area and blocked off by contamination. To count early samples we moved counting equipment from our Apollo, Pennsylvania Uranium Plant.

After decontamination, the exposed technician was released to go home. We supplied him with feces and urine containers and instructed him to collect all excretions. His bioassay data is displayed in Fig. 1.

The next day, we learned that Pittsburgh's Presbyterian-University Hospital had received a thin NaI crystal for its Whole Body Counter. Since this permitted plutonium evaluation, we arranged to have our technician counted that evening.

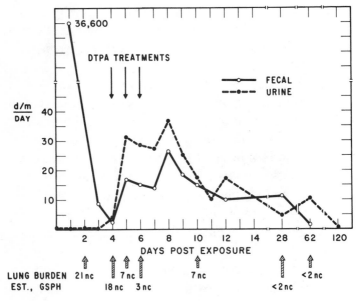

Figure 1.

EXCRETION DATA

ACUTE INHALATION EXPOSURE, January 17, 1966

$^{241}AmO_2$

Because assessing the plutonium burden depended on measuring ^{241}Am and multiplying by the ^{239}Pu to ^{241}Am ratio, the initial estimate of the technician's lung burden was 0.4 μCi. We had assumed a "normal" ratio of 20 to 1. Based on this data, the technician was admitted to the hospital and DTPA was adminis-tered intravenously.

The third day, a sample of the incident contamina-tion was subjected to alpha spectrometry. The actual ^{239}Pu/^{241}Am ratio turned out to be 3/17. This de-creased the burden estimate considerably. However, the DTPA treatment did dramatically increase the urine and feces excretion. By the seventh day, the body burden had fallen to .002 μCi ^{241}Am. The medical aspects of the exposure were discussed by N. Wald and A. Brodsky.[1]

Plant decontamination began the day of the ex-plosion. But, because we had never dealt with such wide spread contamination, much confusion and re-contamination occurred. We had to learn while doing. It took three weeks to complete the decontamination. Later, we were able to handle much worse facility decontamination with relative ease.

2.   PEROXIDE GLOVE BOX EXPLOSION, NOVEMBER 30, 1966

At 2:05 a.m. during a heat "kill", a peroxide filtrate glass tank overpressured and shattered. Two opposing glove box windows blew out, knocking an operator off his feet. Pieces of glass, acting like shrapnel, pierced surrounding glove boxes. ^{239}Pu/^{241}Am contaminated H_2O_2 solution splashed the

operator's face. Exploding glass fragments cut his
right hand.   A helper was standing off to one side and
escaped both injury and serious exposure.

The operator immediately ran to the change room
and showered. He thoroughly washed out his eyes,
saving them from possible peroxide burns. He
showered for ten minutes. Later, the shower hold
tank was assayed at 23 millicuries of ^{239}Pu/^{241}Am.

When the accident occurred, only three operators
and a guard were present. The operator's helper
alerted the guard, who called out emergency personnel.
Health Physics personnel began arriving 35 minutes
after the explosion.

At this time, after long showering, contamination on the operator's face and hands ranged from
250,000 to 2,000,000 c/m/60 cm^2. He was then
wrapped in blankets and placed in a plastic cocoon.
This was very successful in preventing contamination
of the ambulance. While waiting for the ambulance,
Health and Safety personnel washed out the operator's
eyes and bandaged the hand wounds, which were bleeding profusely.

We took the operator to a local hospital, so that
the resident surgeon could examine his injuries. This
had been arranged in our emergency plans. We had
run a training course for doctors and nurses at this
hospital to teach contaminated personnel handling. We
received good cooperation during the incident. The
surgeon sutured the wounds to prevent additional
bleeding. While there, NUMEC Health Physics personnel attempted further decontamination, but only
succeeded in reducing levels by half. It was then
decided to move the patient to Presbyterian-University

Hospital in Pittsburgh, where they were better
equipped to handle the case.

Further decontamination was carried out at the
Presbyterian Hospital morgue. Morgue facilities are
well suited for this kind of contaminated patient
handling. All cleaning fluids are easily saved. Table,
floor and other surfaces are easily cleaned. And the
morgue is usually near an ambulance entrance.

Skin contamination was very stubborn and it took
several days to complete external decontamination.[2]
Shaving all body hair caused a dramatic decrease in
alpha meter readings. The contamination apparently
attached strongly to the hair. A special chelating
concoction finally brought down skin levels.

Body counting data showed possible a high body
burden, so chelation therapy was begun 20 hours after
the accident. Figure 2 shows the operator's gamma
spectrum after 1-1/2 years. The first 24 hours
elimination after DPTA was 1.96×10^5 d/m in the
urine and 3.54×10^6 d/m in the feces.

A NUMEC radiochemist ran a $^{239}Pu/^{241}Am$ ratio
within hours after the explosion. The peroxide solution activity was 25% ^{241}Am. Using this data, the
initial body burden estimate was 0.92 μCi ^{241}Am and
^{239}Pu. Chelation treatments and excision of the hand
wounds helped reduce the burden to about 0.3 μCi.

Although facility contamination was much more
extensive and tenacious, decon efforts were better
organized than for the first accident and it took about
three weeks to restore the plant to normal operation.
We found that personnel traffic must be carefully
controlled to prevent recontamination of cleaned areas.
We used double change lines (and double sets of protective clothing) very successfully in the decontamination.

3. IRIDIUM-192 HOT CELL RELEASE,
JANUARY 13, 1967

NUMEC encapsulates ^{192}Ir sources for radiographic cameras.   The iridium pellets are usually
received in aluminum capsules, which are dissolved
off in caustic solution.

This particular morning, however, the capsules
were of an aluminum alloy and would not dissolve.
The lead Hot Cell technician decided to cut the capsule open.   Without consulting the Hot Cell Engineer,
he set up to make the cut.   It occurred to him that
there was a possibility of contamination release.
So he placed a 2 inch exhaust hose, near the cut off
wheel.   Suction was obtained by using one of the three
cell exhaust ducts.   The technician thought the air
flow through the 2 inch hose would be improved, if
he blocked off the other two exhaust ducts.   So he did.
This action completely eliminated the cell's negative
pressure.

During the cut, the abrasive wheel penetrated the
fuel portion of the capsule.   More than 75 curies were
dispersed in fine particules.   The small diameter hose
exhaust failed completely to capture the high speed
particules generated by the high RPM, cut off wheel.
Figure 3 from the Industrial Ventilation Manual shows
why.   Air velocity falls off rapidly with distance from
the exhaust opening.

The airborne contamination drifted out through the
slave arm manipulators and other cell penetrations.
Completely unaware of the release, the technician
and his helper worked for an hour in the ^{192}Ir cloud.
Only upon leaving for lunch through the change room
and monitoring themselves, did they discover the

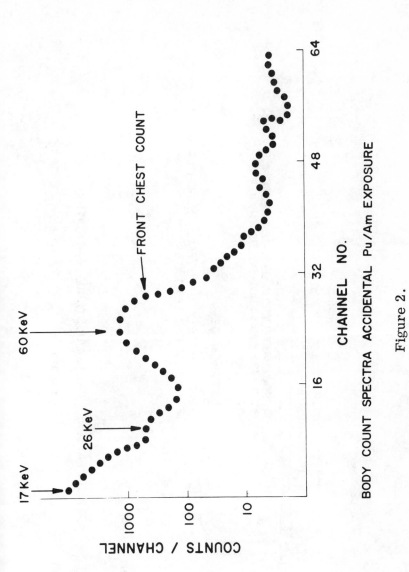

BODY COUNT SPECTRA ACCIDENTAL Pu/Am EXPOSURE

Figure 2.

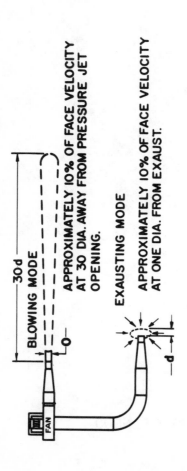

AIR FLOW PATTERNS FROM INDUSTRIAL VENTILATION

Figure 3.

contamination.   They called the Health and Safety
technician, who instructed them to shower.   The fully
protected Health Physics technician made entrance to
the Hot Cell area, found high levels of contamination,
retrieved air samples, and sealed off the cell area
doors with tape.   Although contamination levels were
great enough to generate 20 mR/hr on all horizontal
surfaces, the general air samples did not show corresponding air concentrations.   One hundred and
twenty-five MPC-hours was the maximum exposure
measured at a sampling location.   In light of the
actual cell operator's exposure, the iridium cloud
must have had a very steep concentration gradient.
We have found this sharp disparity in our other
operations by using personal air samplers. [4]

   After showering, the hot cell technicians were
monitored by a Health Physicist.   He noticed gamma
radiation levels of several mR/hr from the chest of
each exposed technician.   There was no appreciable
difference in level when the beta window was closed,
and no contamination could be smeared from the chest
skin.   The Health Physicist concluded that a large
lung deposition had occurred and arranged for body
counting at Presbyterian Hospital.   The deposition
and retention patterns of these cases have been discussed by Brodsky. [5,6]

   To give you some idea of the rather sensational
levels inhaled, both technicians had to be counted
standing outside the body counter to keep the crystal
from jamming, and the first fecal samples measured
20 mR/hr and 8 mR/hr with a gamma survey meter.
The biological half life turned out to be longer than
300 days, but the short physical half life of ^{192}Ir
(74.4 days) limited the lung doses to 45 and 14 rems,

respectively to the lead technician and his helper.
This illustrates an important point: where relative
toxicity is low or half life is short, what might seem
a real "barn burner" of an exposure, nearly always
is less serious than the quieter exposures to ^{239}Pu
or other long lived, highly toxic radionuclides.

Cleaning up the Hot Cell spill proved interesting.
Unlike the alpha activity spills, where, when protected
against inhalation and contamination, recovery personnel may stay indefinitely, we had to control clean up
crews carefully to limit gamma exposure. The Hot
Cell exhaust filters emitted radiation up to 15 R/hr
and were a real problem to change. We managed by
placing shields and writing a detailed procedure for
the change.

The cell interior was much too contaminated for
personnel entry; levels were several hundred R/hr,
even after the intact Ir-192 pellets were shielded.
The first operational problem was unblocking the cell
ducts and restoring negative pressure. This was done,
using the manipulators and a great deal of patience.
Gross cell clean up was done with the manipulators.
When levels reached several R/hour, personnel entry
was possible. Teams for cell entry were organized
from employees with low radiation histories. We
constructed an isolation room at the cell entrance for
outer coverall removal and contamination survey.
Decontamination of the Hot Cell service area was
accomplished in a week, but it was six weeks before
the Hot Cell itself was restored to pre-incident levels.

4. HAND AMPUTATION,
DECEMBER 14, 1967

A technician amputated his right hand while
operating a milling machine in a plutonium glove box.
The accident occurred when the technician's box
glove was caught in the 4 inch cutter tool of a clausing
milling machine, dragging his hand through the cutter.
Figure 4 shows the milling machine. He was reaching past the cutter to adjust an N_2 hose. The hose is
used for blowing chips away from a 3 inch milling
tool, mounted 10 inches back on the same spindle.

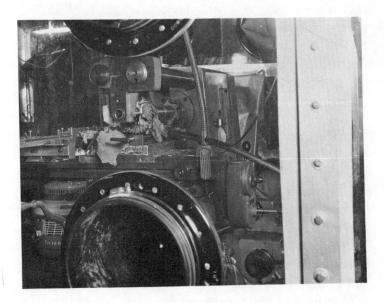

Figure 4.

The milling machine in the glove box
where the amputation occured.

Ordinary procedure called for fixing the N_2 hose while the machine was turned off. The milling machine had been run safely for two years by withdrawing the hands from the glove box and operating the machine with an outside foot switch.

The technician ran some 200 feet to a second floor first aid room. A Health and Safety technician and an engineer applied a tourniquet, stopped the bleeding and called a physician. An alpha survey showed that contamination was limited to the severed wrist.

After receiving medical attention, the technician was transported to Presbyterian Hospital. NUMEC personnel bagged the hand out of the glove box and took it, packed in ice, to the hospital. The hand was decontaminated and grafted back on the arm. About 10 microcuries was estimated by gamma scanning to be left on the hand. Brodsky is reporting separately on the Health Physics evaluation at the hospital.[7] Unfortunately, when warmth failed to return to the hand, it was surgically removed several days later. Less than 0.01 microcuries of plutonium and americium remained in the technician's body, as verified by gamma scanning of the stump, whole body counting and detailed bioassay.

NUMEC Health Physicists deconned the amputated hand. The grossly contaminated hand presented an interesting problem. Since gamma levels from the doubly bagged hand were several mR/hr, we were sure several millicuries of plutonium were inside the bag. We had the hand at the hospital morgue, when the surgeon decided to reattach the hand. A ventilated hood was not available, the contents of the bag were relatively dry and dusty and there was not time to take

the hand to a safe place for cleaning. We solved the
potential radioactive dust problem by injecting saline
solution into the bag and thoroughly wetting the interior. After that, we cut open the bag, without contamination release, and carefully deconned the hand
with surgical soap. Our efforts achieved at least a
factor of 10 reduction in contamination.

No significant release resulted in the Plutonium
Plant. No unusual airborne radioactivity was
measured in the immediate area. Only about 30,000
c/m could be detected on the affected glove port and
this was quickly cleaned up. We found a complete
absence of floor contamination. Although everyone
in the production area was surveyed, we found no one
contaminated, except the wounded technician.

LESSONS LEARNED

Something of value can be retrieved from every
accident. This lesson learned no matter how unimportant it may seem, may be the thing which saves
a life or prevents another accident. Keeping this in
mind, we have listed below some of the things we
have learned from our accidents:

1. Each new operation should be reviewed for
    safe procedures and conditions. This is best
    done by a committee composed of senior tech-
    nical and safety professionals. Even from a
    production viewpoint, it's better to over re-
    view, than possibly omit some important
    point. One accident's lost time and costs
    pays for a lot of review.

2. Nuclear facilities should be compartmentalized
    to reduce the spread of contamination. Where
    a large fabrication area is an absolute neces-
    sity, room ventilation should be controlled so
    that airborne radioactivity does not spread
    contamination throughout a facility.

3. Of course, there should be emergency plans.
    But, some points which may be overlooked
    are:

    a. Telephone numbers and call out lists must
        be constantly updated.

    b. Local hospital personnel must be trained
        in handling contaminated personnel.

    c. Radiation measurements, such as isotope
        ratios, neutron activation analsis, etc,
        which may be used in an emergency, must
        be worked out ahead of time and regularly
        practiced.

    d. There must be a clear delineation of
        authority for post accident situations.
        Otherwise, duplication of effort, crucial
        omissions and working at cross purposes
        occurs.

    e. Radiation instruments must exist in the
        emergency cabinet as well as in the emer-
        gency procedures. You should not count
        on using routine instruments for emer-
        gencies. Too often, they are lost to
        contamination. Emergency instruments
        must be regularly calibrated and main-
        tained. A weekly inspection is not too
        frequent.

f.   Training of emergency personnel must include First Aid. Skill in Health Physics does not guarantee that you know how to stop bleeding or give respiration assistance.

g.   The emergency measurement laboratory and control center locations must be planned to prevent loss of access because of radiation or contamination. You might not be able to improvise, as we did.

4.   Trained, level headed professionals present after an accident are more important than elaborate plans. Every accident we have had has contained some element which we did not foresee. But, thus far, on the spot judgments have been good, and no serious errors have resulted.

5.   The time to beware is when the basic use of a facility changes, as when a solely research laboratory takes on production work. Procedures, equipment, personnel and time scales change so rapidly that conditions for accidents develop.

6.   All safety precautions ordinarily applied to machine tools must be followed when the machinery is in a glove box. In fact, one should be conservative in prescribing safeguards, providing only that the safeguards are not so cumbersome that their use is avoided by operating personnel.

7.   A glove box is a confined volume. A very little flammable material can quickly create

an explosive mixture in a box. Due attention
must be paid to adequate air change rate in
a box, limiting flammable material and providing readily used fire protection.

8. In nearly every accident, the situation initially
appears worse than it really is. If you keep
your head, what appears, at first, to be an
impossible situation will soon become re-
solvable.

REFERENCES

1. N. Wald, A. Brodsky, The Measurement and
Management of Insoluble Plutonium-Americium
Inhalation in Man, IRPA Meeting, Rome, 1966.

2. N. Wald, et. al., Problems in Medical Management of Plutonium-Americium Contaminated
Patients, Symposium on Diagnosis and Treatment of Deposited Radio-nuclides, Richland,
Washington, May 15-17, 1967.

3. Industrial Ventilation, A Manual of Recommended
Practice, 9th ed., American Conference of
Governmental Industrial Hygiensts, 1966.

4. R. Caldwell, T. Potter and E. Schnell, Bioassay
Correlation with Breathing Zone Sampling,
CONF-671048, April, 1968.

5. A. Brodsky, R. Kuhn, I. Sevin and R. Caldwell,
Long Term Clearance of Ir-192 Particulates
from the Human Lung, 14th Annual Bioassay
Meeting, New York, N.Y., October, 1968.

6. A. Brodsky, et. al., Deposition and Retention of ^{192}Ir in the Lung after an Inhalation Incident, Annual Health Physics Meeting, June 1967, Washington, D.C.

7. A. Brodsky, et. al., Americium Contamination Aspects of a Dry Box Incident Involving Hand Amputation, Midyear Symposium Operational Monitoring, Los Angeles, January, 1969.

PLUTONIUM-AMERICIUM CONTAMINATION ASPECTS OF A DRY BOX INVOLVING HAND AMPUTATION*

Allen Brodsky, Sc. D.; Niel Wald, M. D.;
Robert E. Lee, M. D.; John Horm, and
Roger Caldwell
University of Pittsburgh
Presbyterian-University Hospital
Pittsburgh, Pennsylvania

ABSTRACT

An employee whose hand was amputated at the
wrist by a milling machine in a dry box accident was
brought to Presbyterian-University Hospital. About
an hour after he arrived, his contaminated hand was
brought to the hospital and assessed for contamination. Initial counting of the hand indicated high levels
of Pu-Am contamination, which influenced the medical decision regarding rejoining the hand. Several
hours after the patient was brought to the hospital,

---

*This investigation was supported in part by U. S.
Public Health Service Research Grant RH00545-01,
National Center for Radiological Health.

1601

the hand and the stump had been debrided and decontaminated, but there were still hundreds of times the
maximum permissible body burden (based on bone)
of Pu-Am on the hand. However, it was deemed unlikely that very much of the contamination would enter
the blood stream during the anastomosis of blood
vessels and grafting of skin. Thus, the hand was
reattached, but reamputated 3 days later when gan-
grene of the fingers occurred. Further evaluation of
the patient showed that a negligible amount of radioactivity remained on the suture of the stump, the
remaining activity on the stump was removed with the
removal of the remaining scabs, and no measurable
internal burden remained after several weeks. Details of the emergency management are reported,
together with measurements of the distribution of the
remaining contamination on the skin of the hand.

I. INTRODUCTION

On Thursday, December 14, 1967, an employee
whose hand was amputated at the wrist by a milling
machine within a dry box was brought to Presbyterian-
University Hospital. The accident causing the amputation, and health physics operations at the plant,
have been described in the preceding paper of this
conference.[1] This paper will describe the plutonium-
americium contamination problems that influenced
medical decisions and operations at the hospital,
regarding the rejoining of the hand and its reamputation four days later. Since the earliest possible
anastomosis of a severed limb improves chances for
a successful graft, the lessons learned from this

incident may help physicians in future decisions regarding the reattachment of limbs or other operations involving heavy skin contamination. The contamination data may also help in planning of hospital health physics procedures for future incidents.

II. EVENTS PRIOR TO REJOINING THE HAND

Soon after the accident, at about 6:00 p.m., Thursday, December 14, 1967, we received a telephone call at the Radiation Medicine Department of Presbyterian-University Hospital informing us of an accident at a local plutonium processing plant. We were told that an injured employee who was possibly contaminated with plutonium and americium was on his way to the hospital, but we did not know that an amputation was involved. The Technical Director (a health physicist) made several telephone calls and by about 6:15 p.m., the Director (M.D.) was notified that the estimated arrival time of the patient at the hospital was 7-7:15 p.m., and an assistant health physicist and secretary were retained for assistance.

The ambulance containing the patient, driver, and health physics technician arrived at the hospital at 7:00 p.m. and were directed to the morgue entrance leading to our present emergency decontamination facilities, (remote from our low-level whole body counter). The patient was surveyed for external contamination while in the ambulance. No widespread removable alpha activity was found, so the patient was brought in to a decontamination table. We learned that the patient had lost his right hand at the wrist. The patient was relatively calm and cooperative, but

requested a drink of water. Within minutes after the
patient was placed on the table, the medical director
of Radiation Medicine arrived, and the surgeon was
notified. By about 7:15 p.m., the company President
arrived and asked whether the hand had also been
brought to the hospital. He expressed a continued
concern that the hand be reattached immediately.
The assistants who came with the patient said that the
hand had fallen into the contaminated drybox and they
did not know whether it had been removed. At this
time (about 7:30 p.m.), the plant health physics supervisor arrived at the hospital with the contaminated
hand wrapped in plastic in an ice bucket.

The hand was immediately counted with a NaI
crystal while in the ice bucket. The patient was then
dressed in a hospital gown, and rolled on a stretcher
to the whole body counter on the floor above. For
convenience to the patient, doors to the steel room
were opened, our 5" D x 4" NaI crystal, with a 2" D,
5 mil Al, thin window, was moved near the door with
its lower face pointed toward the doorway, and the
patient was placed as shown in Fig. 1 (which was
actually photographed two days later, when the hand
had been rejoined). Spectra such as those in Fig. 2,
compared with our thin 0.13 pCi Am-241 source,
immediately told us (by 8:00 p.m.) that there could
be up to several thousand times the maximum permissible body burden of Pu-Am present, mostly on
the surfaces of the hand and stump. Of course, as
for previous plutonium-incident patients brought to
our hospital,[2,3] we had no definite information on the
Pu/Am activity ratio for the first few hours, but
could see some evidence of the additional "17-kev"
L x-rays of plutonium daughters (Figs. 2-4). An

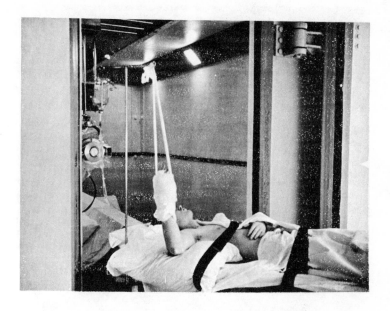

Fig. 1.   Picture of Patient with Rejoined Hand and Forearm Raised at 47 inches from 5"D x 4" NaI Crystal Having 2" Thin Window, December 16, 1967.

initial estimate from the company president indicated that the material handled in the drybox contained 600 ppm americium, or an Am-241/Pu alpha activity ratio of about 0.032.   This ratio was used to initially estimate that the total contamination on the hand and stump might be up to perhaps several tens of thousands of times the maximum permissible bone burdens of the Pu-Am mixture.

In order to save time while the patient's stump was being counted, the hand was immediately taken (about 8:00 p. m.) from the whole body counter to

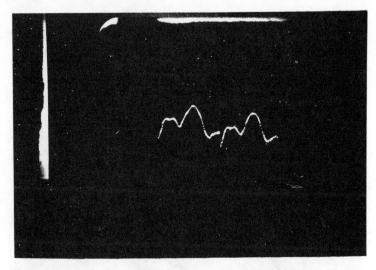

Fig. 2.   Comparison of 10 Minute Spectra of
Hand and Stump on December 14, 1967.

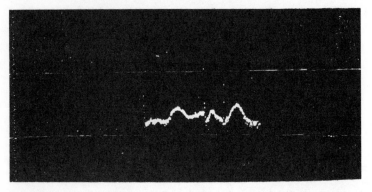

Fig. 3.   Left: Spectrum of Patient's Reattached
Hand at 47 inches from 5"D x 4" Crystal as in Fig.
1.   Right: Spectrum of 1 Liter Solution of 0.06 μCi
Am-241 in Bottle Against 5" D x 4" Crystal, December 16, 1967.   Note the attenuation of the 17
kev portion of the spectrum from the hand by the
thick bandage.

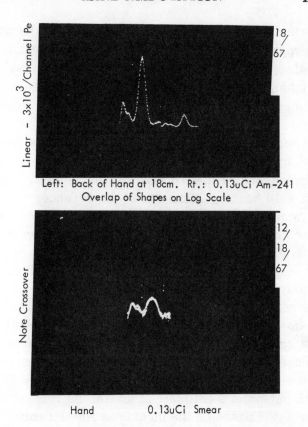

Fig. 4. Comparison of Spectra of Hand on
December 18, 1967, after Reamputation (left)
and Thin Am-241 Source (right), on Both Linear
(top) and Logarithmic (bottom) Count/Channel
Scales. (In bottom picture, display is in over-
lap mode and vertically superimposed to show
similar relative intensities of "17 kev" and
60 kev spectral regions. Without the bandage,
and a slight reduction of the air attenuation, the
17 kev portion of the spectrum from the hand
reappears.

decontaminate it*, debride the tissues near the wrist,
and prepare the hand for possible reattachment.
Counting information was given to the physicians as it
was taken so they could continuously weigh the possible risks of an internal body burden of Pu-Am versus
the possible benefits of reattaching the hand. Chances
for a successful hand graft were estimated as about
5-10% by the surgeon, with the probability of success
likely decreasing toward zero for any delay beyond
about 9-10 hours. Time was of the essence.

Additional measurements were obtained on the
cleaned and debrided hand, and the debridements from
the patient's stump (it was inadvisable and unnecessary
to move the patient again to the whole body counter).
No early urinalyses were available but gross counts
of excreta and the nature of the incident indicated
that any internal body burden was at this time insignificant compared to the quantities of activity on skin
surfaces. Cleaning and debriding the hand had lowered
surface contamination to about 10 μCi based on the
health physicist's estimate of an Am/Pu ratio of 0.1
(later 4 μCi based on the measured Am/Pu ratio
obtained at 3:30 a.m., December 15, 1967); debridements from the stump contained only about 20% of the
activity that had been on the stump (see Table 1). The
remaining contamination on the hand and stump was
still more than one hundred times the MPBB. However, the contamination was believed to be relatively
fixed on the skin surface. At 12:40 a.m., Friday,
December 15, 1967, the decision was made to reattach the hand, and the surgeon proceeded to the
operating room, where preparations for the

---

*Surgical soap, pHisohex, was used.

Table 1
SEQUENCE OF CONTAMINATION MEASUREMENTS ON HAND AND ARM

TIME AND DATE	SITUATION	TOTAL ALPHA ACTIVITY	
		IMMEDIATE ESTIMATE	FINAL ESTIMATE*
8:00-8:40 p.m., Thurs., 12/14/67 (2 HOURS POST ACCIDENT)	HAND (SEVERED)	300 µCi*	100 µCi
	STUMP (BEFORE DEBRIDEMENT)	40 µCi* (TOTAL >10,000 MPBB)	5 µCi (TOTAL >4,000 MPBB)
12:40 a.m., Fri., 12/15/67 (7 HOURS POST ACCIDENT)	HAND (SEVERED)	10 µCi*	4 µCi
	STUMP (AFTER DEBRIDEMENT)	10 µCi* (TOTAL >100 MPBB)	4 µCi (TOTAL >100 MPBB)
Sat., 12/16/67 (2 DAYS POST ACCIDENT)	HAND AND STUMP (REJOINED, 1:30-5:30 a.m., Fri., 12/15/67)	9 µCi TOTAL	9 µCi TOTAL
Mon., 12/18/67 (4 DAYS POST ACCIDENT)	HAND (REAMPUTATED)	4 µCi	4 µCi
	NEW STUMP (AMPUTATION - 3:00 p.m., 12/18/67)	0.009 µCi	0.009 µCi
Tues., 1/30/68 (1 1/2 MONTHS POST ACCIDENT)	STUMP, AFTER REMOVING MOST CONTAMINATED SCAB	FINAL ALPHA ACTIVITY REMOVED WITH SUTURES AND SURFACE SCABS	
	TOTAL BODY	NO ACTIVITY DETECTABLE (< 0.002 µCi)	

*Initial estimates based on Am/Pu activity ratio of only 0.032 - 0.1; final estimates based on an average Am/Pu alpha activity ratio of about 1:3 for materials in drybox at time of accident, determined at 3:30 a.m., 12/15/67.

operation were already underway. About 1 1/2 hours
had been required to evaluate the unprecedented re-
contamination problem and arrive at a medical decision. Most of the radioactivity measurements and
evaluations were carried out concurrently with other
preparations for the operation.

III. CONTAMINATION LEVELS WITH
HAND REJOINED

At 1:30 a.m., December 15, about 8 hours after
the accident, the hand was perfused with saline and
DTPA solution. Also, 1 gram DTPA was administered
intravenously to the patient to immediately chelate
any Pu or Am that might enter the system, and the
rejoining operation began. Surgeons were instructed
to retain for later survey any instruments coming
into contact with the contamination, and to discard
any wastes that might be contaminated for disposal in
a plastic bag. Health physicists observed the operation from a balcony. The main arteries and veins of
the hand and arm were rejoined and blood flow was
restored to the hand. The operation was completed
about 5:30 a.m., and from about 6:30-7:30 a.m.,
health physicists from the plant and the University
collected wastes and checked the operating room.
Wastes were shipped to the company, slightly contaminated surgical instruments were sent to the
University Radiation Safety Office for decontamination
(which turned out to be successful), and the operating
room was approved for routine use within a few hours.
None of the hospital or surgical staff was found to be
contaminated.

On Saturday, December 16, 1967, the patient was taken to the whole body counter and the reattached hand and arm were counted again, as shown in Fig. 1. Spectra were corrected for body potassium and background contributions by shielding the hand itself to obtain control counts. Figure 2 shows, on the left, a spectrum of the patient's reattached hand at 47 inches from the 5" D x 4" crystal. On the right for comparison is the spectrum of the 0.06 μCi dissolved in 1 liter of solution. The net self-absorption of the 60-kev peak for equivalent amounts of tissue mass would be negligible.[4] However, the appreciable attenuation of the "17 kev" x-ray group by the relatively thick bandage and brace is evident in the left-hand spectrum. This illustrates the advantage of using the 60-kev Am-241 peak for quantitation when it is present in sufficient abundance. As shown in Table 1 by the results at 2 days post accident, the total contamination was not reduced appreciably by the rejoining (anastomosis) operation.

IV. CONTAMINATION AFTER REAMPUTATION

Unfortunately, circulation in the fingertips of the hand did not improve quickly enough, and the hand was reamputated at 3:00-3:10 p.m., Monday, December 18, 1967. The hand was infused with formaldehyde and recounted after amputation, showing about 4 μCi Pu-Am distributed over the surface. In Fig. 4, spectra of the hand without the bandage are shown on the left (top and bottom); and spectra of a thin Am-241 source are shown on the right. The prominent 17 kev peak from that contamination on the side of the hand toward the detector, and the similarity in shape and magnitude between spectra (not shown) from the back and front of the hand, indicated that the major part, if not all, of the contamination of the hand still remained distributed on the surface. Since the reamputation of the hand was done approximately an inch higher than the original accidental amputation, the reamputated hand turned out to contain practically all of the remaining contamination.

On Tuesday, December 19, 1967, the patient was brought to the whole body counter and the activity remaining in the stump was measured (see Fig. 5). In Fig. 6, the spectrum from the stump (left) at 17 cm below the 5" D x 4" crystal showed only 0.0088 μCi Am-241 remaining; at the same time, the spectrum of the 8" D x 4" crystal against the patient's back showed no appreciable (< 0.002 μCi) lung or systemic burden.[5] After the first two days, no Pu-Am activity was found in the urine, so either no contamination had entered the system, or whatever amount entered was immediately removed by the DTPA. Further measurements with alpha detectors were made when the patient returned to Dr. Niemann's office for removal of sutures and inspection of the healing skin. These surveys located alpha activity extremely close to the surface, which was completely removed with the last scab on Tuesday, January 30, 1968 (1 1/2 months post accident). Further whole body counter measurements detected no remaining activity in or on the body (see Table 1).

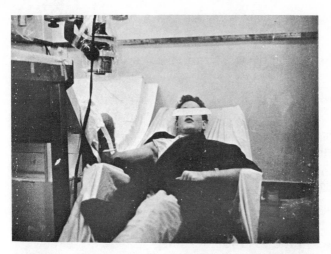

Fig. 5. Photograph of Patient in Lawn Chair,
with Stump 17 cm Below Window of 5" D x 4"
Crystal, December 19, 1967.

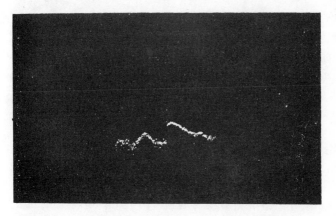

Fig. 6. Left: Spectrum from Stump as in Position in Fig. 5, Indicating only 0.0088 μCi Am-241
in Surface Scabs. Right: Spectrum of 8" D x 4"
Crystal Behind Back, Showing No Appreciable
Systemic Am-241.

V. EXAMINATION OF THE AMPUTATED HAND

After the reamputated hand was counted (Fig. 4),
it was preserved in a 2-liter bottle of formaldehyde
for further examination. On Febrary 14, 1968, the
skin was dissected from the hand (only 0.006 μCi was
on the pathologist's glove after this procedure). A
special collimator was constructed having a square
window and the skin from the front and back of the
hand was scanned in squares with the apparatus shown
in Fig. 7. Figures 8 and 9 show photographs of the
skin from the front and back of the hand, respectively,
placed in the grid for scanning. Figure 10 shows a
summary of the net counts/minute of the 2" x 1mm
NaI crystal looking through the collimator. A similar
distribution of activity was found on the back of the
hand.

Concentrations of contamination were particularly
high near the edges where the skin had been sutured
together, and near the back knuckles, as shown also
by an alpha survey. Alpha counts on the skin of the
hand after it had been in the formaldehyde were
generally about several thousand counts/minute per
100 cm^2 with the Eberline PAC-4G held about 1 1/2
cm from the surface, but peaks up to 50,000 counts/
minute per 100 cm^2 were obtained near the sutures.
Remarkably, both the inside and outside surfaces of
the skin, palm and back, gave in each case about
equal alpha activity, indicating that the formaldehyde
had probably transferred contamination through the
skin.

Unfortunately, the hand (after skinning) was in-
advertently placed back in the contaminated formaldehyde (as a result of inadequate briefing and/or written

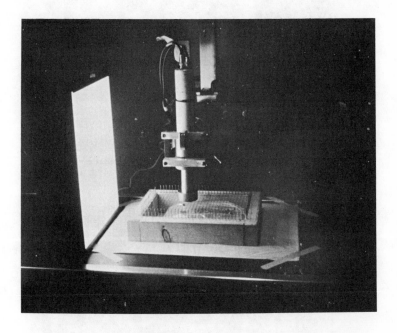

Fig. 7. Apparatus for Examining Distribution
of Americium on Surface of Skin - 2″ D × 1mm
NaI Crystal Looking Through Brass Collimator
at Rectangular Position of Grid.

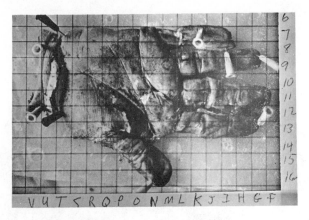

Fig. 8. Photograph of Skin Removed from Palm of Hand and Grid System for Defining Locations of Measurements.

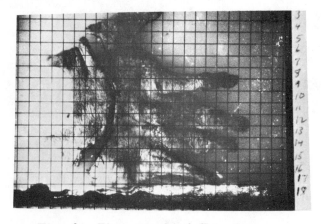

Fig. 9. Photograph of Skin from Back of Hand, and Coordinates of Grid for Measurements Over Skin of Front of Hand.

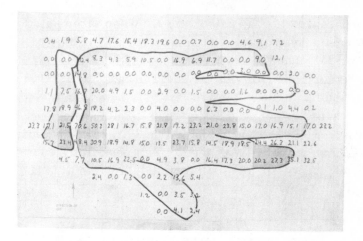

Fig. 10a. Summary of Relative X-Ray Count
Seen Through a Collimator Over Various Portions of the Palm, Showing the Wide Distribution of Contamination on the Hand.

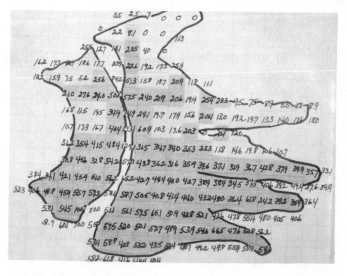

Fig. 10b. Net Counts/minute—back of hand.

procedures for the pathologist). When taken out of the formaldehyde again, the hand contained about 1 μCi Am-241 plus Pu, so it was impossible to determine whether alpha activity transferred through the skin by the formaldehyde was also distributed throughout the hand. When soaked in fresh formaldehyde for two days, the contaminated hand transferred only 0.0044 μCi Am-241 (0.44%) of the activity back to the formaldehyde. Also, the original formaldehyde solution had retained only 0.0535 μCi.

VI. SUMMARY AND CONCLUSIONS

The patient's contamination levels before and after each operation have been summarized in Table 1. The following conclusions may be derived from this incident:

1. Limbs grossly contaminated (on the surface only) with hundreds of MPBB, Pu or Am, may be reattached after careful cleaning and debridement without appreciable risk of internal exposure for at least several days after reattachment.

2. Surgical and counting operations may be carried out at practically no risk to hospital personnel or equipment, with appropriate health physics supervision and instructions.

3. Since no systemic burden remained in the patient, it appears likely that formaldehyde may carry Pu-Am contamination as it diffuses through tissues. Thus, any tissue

samples for further radioactivity studies should be taken and sectioned before preservation in formaldehyde.

REFERENCES

1. Roger Caldwell, Thomas Potter, and Edward Schnell, "Radiological Emergency Experience in an Industrial Plutonium Plant," Presented at the Health Physics Society Midyear Symposium, January 28-31, 1969.

2. N. Wald, R. Wechsler, A. Brodsky and S. Yaniv, "Problems in Independent Medical Management of Plutonium-Americium Contaminated Patients", in "Proceedings of a Symposium on Diagnosis and Treatment of Deposited Radionuclides", May 15-17, 1967, Edited by H. A. Kornberg and W. D. Norwood, 1968.

3. A. Brodsky, J. A. Sayeg, N. Wald, R. Wechsler, and R. Caldwell, "The Measurement and Management of Insoluble Plutonium-Americium Inhalation in Man," in "Proceedings of the First International Congress of Radiation Protection, Sept. 5-10, 1966," Edited by W. S. Snyder, H. H. Abee, L. K. Burton, R. Maushart, A. Benco, F. Duhamel, and B. M. Wheatley, Pergamon Press, 1968, Vol. 2, pp. 1181-1190.

4. A. G. Bukovitz, J. A. Sayeg, A. A. Spritzer, and A. Brodsky, "Effective Transmission of the Human Thorax for Photons from ^{239}Pu, ^{241}Am, and Other Low-Energy Emitters," in press, Health Physics, 1969.

5. These NaI crystals and geometries have
    essentially been calibrated by the long-term
    follow-up of a patient having an initial 2 μCi
    Am-241 body burden, mostly in bone and liver.
    (A. Brodsky and N. Wald, "Removal of Am-241
    from a Human Case by Chelation Therapy," pre-
    sented at the 14th Annual Bioassay Meeting,
    sponsored by the Health and Safety Laboratory,
    U.S. Atomic Energy Commission, New York,
    N.Y., October 8, 1968.)

PROMPT HANDLING OF CASES INVOLVING ACCIDENTAL EXPOSURE TO PLUTONIUM

K. R. Heid and J. J. Jech
Battelle Memorial Institute
Pacific Northwest Laboratory
Richland, Washington

ABSTRACT

Accidents involving exposure, or potential for exposure, to plutonium require prompt analysis and action by trained radiation protection and medical personnel to facilitate rapid evaluation of the seriousness of the exposure and possible therapeutic treatment to minimize ultimate deposition within the body. Procedures used at Hanford to screen, evaluate and report accidents are briefly described. The types of data collected to aid in these evaluations are discussed. The effectiveness of these procedures based on the experience of approximately 2000 plutonium workers over a 23-year span is reviewed. Studies in progress to improve capabilities for initiating prompt mitigatory action are briefly discussed.

1621

INTRODUCTION

With the increasing use of radionuclides in industry, prompt mitigatory action following accidental exposure to plutonium assumes greater importance. This is primarily true because of its extremely long life and selective deposition within the body. This paper is based on 46,000 man years of plutonium work at Hanford which has included a variety of manufacturing and R & D programs and has involved several isotopes and chemical forms of plutonium. During this period there have been roughly 1370 cases at Hanford involving accidental exposures to plutonium which have required investigation (Tables 1 and 2). Of these - 1% of the cases resulted in depositions ≥ 50% of the MPBB of 40 nCi using bone as reference however, about one out of five resulted in some kind of internal deposition.

CHELATING AGENTS

The chelate usually administered is a solution of the trisodium-calcium salt of diethylenetriamine-pentaacetic acid (DTPA). If a significant quantity of plutonium is found in the wound or is suspected, based on early survey measurements, DTPA may be administered prior to completion of decontamination efforts or concurrently with the surgical removal of the contaminant. If the contaminant appears to have been soluble or if prudence dictates discontinuance of surgical excision before the contaminant has been totally removed, the wound may be flushed using DTPA solution before the excised area is closed. In cases where the potential for internal deposition of a significant quantity of plutonium seems minimal, as is indicated by the amount of plutonium measured in the wound prior to excision and the length of exposure,

Table 1.

Plutonium Contaminated Injuries At Hanford:
1946 Through 1967

	Number of Cases	Per Cent of Total
Injury cases potentially contaminated	230	100
Cases containing measurable plutonium contamination	136	59
Cases surgically decontaminated	86	37
Cases resulting in plutonium deposition $\geqslant 5\%$ MPBB	15	6.5
Cases resulting in plutonium deposition $\geqslant 50\%$ MPBB	5	2

the amount remaining in the wound after excision and the probable solubility of the contaminant; the physician may decide to wait for assay results of rush processed urine samples before deciding whether or not to administer DTPA. Continuation of DTPA treatment will depend upon several factors, one of which is the effectiveness of the treatment indicated by the rate of increase of plutonium excreted in the urine. Therefore, urine samples are collected and processed daily to keep the physician informed of the apparent effectiveness of the treatments and the desirability for continuing treatment.

If available data suggest that the systemic deposition may exceed 0.01 μCi ^{239}Pu, a temporary work restriction precluding further work with plutonium or other biologically similar radionuclides will be issued until a complete evaluation can be completed. Close liaison between radiation protection and medical personnel will be necessary for several weeks, months, or even years post intake in extreme cases.

INTAKE VIA INHALATION

If the mode of intake is known or suspected to be inhalation, an early evaluation of the internally deposited plutonium is more difficult. The detection of plutonium on protective clothing, skin, nasal smears, nose blows, sputum samples, work area surfaces, and air samples are usually the first indicators that inhalation may have occurred. Any skin contamination is quickly removed to the extent possible using mild reagents initially and progressively stronger reagents as needed. Nasal passages, if contaminated, are irrigated with normal saline solution. The irrigation process may be repeated several times if necessary to reduce the nasal contamination. Eyes, if contaminated, are flushed, using tap water. Efforts are made to decontaminate skin surfaces to < 500 d/m and nasal passages until smears and/or nose blows contain < 50 d/m—provided the time required will not jeopardize the effectiveness of therapeutic treatment. Decontamination should not be continued to the extent that the skin becomes tender or is damaged so that subsequent absorption into the blood stream could occur. On the contrary, personnel

Table 2.

Plutonium Inhalation Cases at Hanford:
1946 Through 1967

	Number of Cases	Per Cent of Total
Plutonium inhalation cases	1140	100
Cases treated with chelating agent	12	1
Cases resulting in plutonium deposition ⩾ 5% MPBB	98	9
Cases resulting in plutonium deposition ⩾ 50% MPBB	12	1

may be released while still contaminated provided the contaminant is fixed and covered to prevent any possible spread. Further decontamination can be performed later as skin conditions permit. The radiation protection representative at the site will then quickly collect supporting data that may be available such as an estimate of the duration of the exposure to the contaminated atmosphere; the concentration of contamination in the air; the chemical and physical form of the plutonium involved; a sample of the contaminant such as a smear of contaminated skin surface, preferably facial contamination, if available; a sample of the contaminant as collected on nasal smears, in a nose blow, or in sputum samples; and a single voiding sample of urine. A listing of types of data collected is shown in Table 3. Based upon

Table 3.

Types of Data Which May be Collected
for Plutonium Inhalation Incidents

1. Urine analysis

2. Feces analysis

3. In-vivo examination

4. Isotopic composition and Pu alpha/^{241}Am alpha ratio

5. Chemical form of the aerosol

6. Solubility of the aerosol

7. Particle size (air samples—nasal smears)

8. Nasal and skin contamination activity

9. Concentration of plutonium aerosol

10. Duration of exposure

11. Other details of incident

the preliminary information provided by the field radiation protection personnel, the exposure evaluator will make initial estimates as to the probable severity of the intake. Depending upon the apparent severity, he will make arrangements for a lung counter examination, provide liaison with medical personnel for possible therapeutic treatment, and arrange for the collection of whatever additional data may be useful in evaluating the intake. This will usually include the collection and analysis of the various samples collected

such as urine, feces, and possibly blood samples.
He will also schedule additional lung counter examinations, if appropriate.

The initial evaluation of the extent of the intake
is most useful if available within the first few hours.
If the initial evaluation indicates a high probability for
inhalation of plutonium, an industrial physical will
decide if treatment is advisable. Treatment may
include inhalation of a lung irritant with a nebulizer
to induce coughing and hopefully speed up clearance
from the upper respiratory tract and/or administration of DTPA.

LATER ACTION FOR INHALATION CASES

For those inhalation cases where DTPA is administered, follow-up treatments may be scheduled
if deemed warranted by occupational medical personnel. As in the injury case, continuation of DTPA
treatment is dependent on its apparent effectiveness
as indicated by results of rush analysis of 100 ml
aliquots of urine samples which are collected daily
while treatment is being administered.

Follow-up lung counter examinations are made as
considered necessary for evaluation purposes. Examinations made at day 7 to 10 post-intake, immediately following the rapid lung clearance phase, are
of the utmost importance. The results from these
and subsequent examinations are utilized to make
evaluations based on the concepts in the new lung
model.[5,6] Where possible frequent examinations are
scheduled during the early phase clearance period
(first seven days post-intake) to obtain data relevant
to early clearance rates. These later data are

obtained primarily for special study purposes and may
occasionally be difficult to obtain due to the reluct-
ance of management to restrict employees from work
for such study.

The collection of urine and fecal samples are also
important for evaluation purposes. The basis upon
which these samples and lung counter examinations
are scheduled at Hanford are defined in Table 4.

The initial fecal samples are analyzed by gamma
ray spectrometry techniques to determine the ^{241}Am
content. Provided the Pu/Am ratio is known or can
be obtained, a crude estimate of the severity of the
intake may be made based on ^{241}Am content in these
fecal samples. Fecal samples for the first 5 days
post-intake are analyzed both for plutonium and americium. The americium data are used for comparison
to earlier gamma spectrometry data and as an aid in
establishing the Pu/Am ratio. The plutonium data
are used for making evaluations based on the new lung
model concepts. Delayed fecal samples (t ≥ 7 days
post intake) are scheduled coincident with lung counter
examinations. The delayed fecal data are used to
estimate the pulmonary burden based upon the slow-
clearance from the pulmonary to the G.I. tract. As
reported by Caldwell[7] an excretion rate of 1 pCi/day
indicates a corresponding pulmonary burden of 1 nCi
of relatively insoluble plutonium. This relation is
useful for comparison to and in support of lung counter
examination data. Evaluations from early fecal data
and lung counter examination data are made applying
the techniques described earlier.[6]

Additional data are necessary to complete the
evaluations from lung counter examination data and
fecal data. These include primarily particle size,

Table 4.

Criteria for Scheduling Feces Samples

Schedule No. 1

Obtain Five Daily Fecal Samples Within the First Seven Days Post Intake

A. Nasal smears exceed 500 d/m

B. Nasal smears > 100 < 500 d/m and exposure duration ≫ 5 min.

C. Nasal smears > 5 < 100 d/m and exposure duration > 30 min.

D. Exposure to fumes from a fire

E. Air sample results exceed 2 x 10^{-10} μCi/cc for an 8-hour period and exposure duration > 1 hour

Schedule No. 2

Obtain One Fecal Sample On the Second Day Post Intake

A. Nasal smears are positive but do not meet criteria in schedule No. 1

B. Any other person in the same incident meets the criteria in schedule No. 1

C. Air sample results exceed 2 x 10^{-11} μCi/cc for an 8-hour period

D. Widespread skin contamination a dry form or facial contamination > 1000 d/m

E. Clothing contamination a dry form > 5000 d/m

Table 4 (cont.)

F.   Possible plutonium inhalation is suspected
     for other reasons

Schedule No. 3
    Obtain Two Fecal Samples at Periods > 10 Days
Post Incident

A.   Obtain samples to coincide with positive lung
     counter examinations preferably following
     two days off of work on the 15th and 30th days
     post intake. Schedule at approximately
     monthly intervals thereafter provided that
     data useful for evaluations are obtained.

---

solubility, isotopic composition and the Pu/Am ratio
of the plutonium involved. Particle size information
is obtained for nasal and skin smears and for a sample
of the contaminant collected on an air sample filter.
Smears of nasal and skin contamination are also used
to obtain data regarding solubility and isotopic composition. Particle size and isotopic composition data
are obtained using the techniques defined by
Anderson.[8, 9, 10] The isotopic composition data are
necessary to determine the Pu/Am ratio and to establish the ^{241}Pu content. The Pu/Am ratio is vital for
evaluating lung counter examination data since the
technique used at Hanford involves the measurement
of the 60 keV photon from ^{241}Am.[11, 12] It is vital
that this ratio be firmly established since false or
inaccurate assumptions will be very misleading.
Knowledge of ^{241}Pu content is essential at Hanford
since it is a beta emitter and separate calculations
are made to determine the additional deposition resulting from the isotope.[13] It is also essential to

predict the ^{241}Am growth and effect on lung counter examinations.

Although early survey data, lung counter examination data and fecal data are used for initial, early, and intermediate evaluation; the final complete evaluations of the systemic deposition of plutonium are based on urine data. The systemic deposition of initially soluble plutonium is evaluated using early urine data and the Langham Model[14] while the deposition of initially insoluble plutonium is evaluated from delayed urine data and the Healy Model.[15] The evaluations made by the above techniques are collected, compared and correlated as a part of a long range study being conducted at Hanford.

Data from an actual inhalation case may be of interest when examined in detail. Figure 1 shows the data obtained for a case in which the lung count data followed the predictions of the lung model and in which the deposition estimates based on fecal and lung count data agrees reasonably well. In this case, the employee incurred plutonium oxide facial and nasal contamination of 20 nCi when he failed to attach a cannister to his face mask. The exposure duration was 20 minutes and analysis of the material on filter sampler showed an original Pu/Am ratio of 13, a ^{241}Pu weight percent of 0.4, and a particle size of 7μ (AMAD). * The employee had no previous history of internally deposited plutonium and did not return to plutonium work during the collection of these data. Projection of the lung counter examination data for the slow clearance phase to time zero gives an intercept value of 11 nCi which is 0.6 of the initial pulmonary deposition. Therefore, an initial pulmonary deposition of 18 nCi is indicated as compared to 11 nCi when based on fecal data. The slope of the curve

*Activity mean aerodynamic diameter

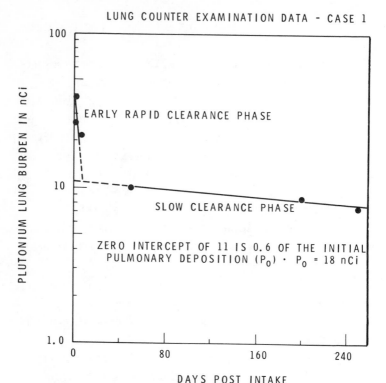

Fig. 1. Lung Counter Examination Data for Case 1—Inhalation of Plutonium Oxide Having an Initial Ratio of $^{239}Pu/^{241}Am$ of 13 and 0.4 Wt% of ^{241}Pu.

indicates a clearance rate equivalent to a 500 day half-life. Delayed fecal data indicates a lung burden of 10 nCi on day 200 which agreed well with the lung count value of 9 nCi. Estimates of the ultimate systemic deposition are 2 nCi based on feces and 3 nCi based on lung counter examination data. These may be compared to a systemic burden of 6 nCi based on evaluation of urine data.

GUIDES FOR INITIAL AND EARLY
ASSESSMENTS OF INHALATION CASES

Data obtained to date from plutonium oxide inhalation cases for long-range study purposes provide some correlations which may be useful as guides in making initial estimates. It is emphasized that these correlation guides are used at Hanford only to make an initial estimate as an aid for determining prompt mitigatory action. The correlations established are based on initial nasal smear data which, in most instances, are probably the best indicator of severity of intake from early survey data. Judgment should be used in applying these guides since incident details such as (1) abnormal particle sizes such as may be associated with fires and explosion; (2) breathing habits of the exposed persons (mouth breathers); (3) cross contamination of nasal smears from lips or facial contamination, may cause large variance from these correlations. The correlations and guides have been established for plutonium oxide cases only. Final and formal evaluations should be based upon bioassay data using established models and upon lung counter examination data where available.

Correlations between nasal smear activity and early fecal data and/or estimates of depositions calculated from early fecal data are shown on Figs. 2 and 3. For most of the cases at Hanford, as indicated in Fig. 2, five times the nasal smear activity may be used as an approximation of the activity in the early fecal exretion (total excretion from the first 5 days post intake). The correlation shown on Fig. 3

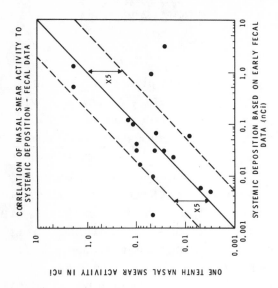

Fig. 3. Comparison of Nasal Smear Activity to Systemic Deposition Based on Early Fecal Data and ICRP Task Group II Lung Model Concepts—for Plutonium Oxide Inhalation Cases

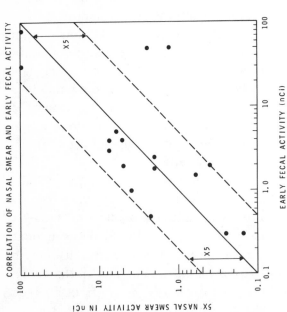

Fig. 2. Comparison of Nasal Smear Activity to Early Fecal Data—for Plutonium Oxide Inhalation Cases

indicates that 1/10 of the nasal smear activity is equivalent to the systemic deposition as calculated from early fecal data. The data presented in Figs. 1 and 2 appear to correlate within a factor of five. These correlations have been extended further using Lung Model Concepts to relate nasal smear activity to lung burdens. These relationships have been determined for inhalation of plutonium oxide aerosols having a particle size of 4μ (AMAD) since this appears to be the mean particle size in the majority of Hanford incident cases. These relationships, which are shown as guides in Fig. 4, indicate that for an initial nasal smear of 1 nCi, systemic and initial pulmonary burdens of 0.1 nCi and 1.0 nCi respectively may represent reasonable early estimates. Although these were established from the relationship between nasal smear and early fecal data, reasonable confirmation has been obtained in many of these cases with estimates based on lung counter examination data.

For facilities which have lung counter examination capability, the problems in making initial estimates are minimized. At Hanford we use the guides shown in Fig. 5 to make initial assessments based on early lung count data for oxide inhalation cases. These guides were established assuming a 4μ particle size. However, a broader range to cover the particle size range of interest, can be readily established from the lung model concepts. For initial assessment purposes, the guides established for 4μ particles are normally adequate. The guides given on Fig. 5 indicate the assumed plutonium intake associated with an initial lung count examination result of 1/nCi of ^{241}Am.

The data presented in Figs. 4 and 5 should be used cautiously since they were developed only as an

Nasal Smear	Initial Pulmonary Burden	Pulmonary Burden at t = 7 days	Initial Lung Burden	Ultimate Systemic Burden
1 nCi	1 nCi	0.6 nCi	3 nCi	0.1 nCi

Note:

1. The above data are based on 30 plutonium oxide inhalation cases at Hanford. Relationships are derived from initial nasal smear data that were obtained using extreme care to prevent cross contamination from lip or facial contamination and from evaluations of depositions using early facal data, lung counter examination data and the new ICRP Lung Model Concepts.

2. The correlations made appear to be valid within a factor of $\pm$ 5; however, estimates obtained using these correlations should be used only as an aid in determining prompt mitigatory action.

Fig. 4. Guide for Estimating Internal Deposition Based On Nasal Smear Data—Pu Oxide, 4 µ Particle.

Initial Lung Count-241 Am	Initial Lung Burden - Pu	Pulmonary Burden-Pu Initial	Pulmonary Burden-Pu t=7 days	Resultant System Burden - Pu
1 nCi	15 nCi	5 nCi	3 nCi	0.5 nCi

Note: Estimates obtained using data in this guide should be used only as an aid in determining prompt mitigatory action.

Fig. 5. Guide For Estimating Internal Deposition Based On Lung Counter Data—Pu/Am Ratio = 15.

aid for making very early assessments of the probable
severity of plutonium inhalation cases. The care used
in obtaining nasal smears, the possibility that a person might be a mouth breather, deposition resulting
from incidents involving fires and explosions, should
all be carefully considered before the guides are
applied.

REFERENCES

1. W. D. Norwood, "Removal of Plutonium and
    Other Transuranic Elements from Man". Paper
    presented at the International Atomic Energy
    Agency/World Health Organization Scientific
    Meeting on Diagnosis of Treatment of Radioactive
    Poisoning.

2. E. D. Dyson and S. A. Beach, Health Physics
    Vol. 15, 385-397 (1968).

3. K. R. Heid, R. C. Henle and J. M. Selby,
    "Prompt Mitigatory Action After Accidental Ex-
    Posure to Radionuclides", BNWL-SA-962 (1967).

4. R. J. Epstein and E. W. Johanson, Health Physics
    Vol. 12, 29-35 (1966).

5. ICRP Task Group on Lung Dynamics, Health
    Physics Vol. 12, 173 (1966).

6. K. R. Heid, J. J. Jech, "Assessing the Probable
    Severity of Plutonium Inhalation Cases", BNWL-
    SA-1595 (1968).

7. R. Caldwell, "The Detection of Insoluble Alpha
    Emitters in the Lung",   unpublished.

8. B. V. Andersen, Health Physics Vol. 10, 899-907 (1964).

9. B. V. Andersen, P. E. Bramson and H. V. Larson, "Supplementary Data Sources for Evaluation of Insoluble Actinide Inhalation Exposures", BNWL-SA-1572 (1968).

10. B. V. Andersen and I. C. Nelson, "Plutonium Air Concentrations and Particle Size Relationships in Hanford Facilities", BNWL-495, (1967).

11. M. R. Boss and J. R. Mann, Health Physics Vol. 13, 259-266 (1967).

12. B. V. Andersen, P. E. Bramson and H. V. Larson, "Dosimetry of Alpha Emitters in the Lung", BNWL-SA-1765 (1968).

13. K. R. Heid, unpublished data.

14. W. H. Langham, Amer. Ind. Hyg. Assoc. 17, 305-318 (1956).

15. J. W. Healy, Amer. Ind. Hyg. Assoc. 18, 261-266 (1957).

Session X
COMMUNICATIONS AND MANAGEMENT

Chairman

FRANK O. BOLD
Gulf General Atomics
San Diego, Calif.

T^{2}WR
(THINK, TALK, WRITE AND REASON)

Carl M. Unruh
Battelle Memorial Institute
Pacific Northwest Laboratory
Richland, Washington

ABSTRACT

The ability to communicate all levels of knowledge
is one of man's unique abilities. To use this ability
to have good communications requires one to think,
talk, write and reason. The health physicist, if he is
to be effective in his profession, needs to develop his
communication capabilities with craftsmen, management, and the public. He can accomplish his necessary work only through effective thinking, talking,
writing and reasoning. His communications should
meet the needs of and be understood by those receiving them.

Second only to a thorough knowledge of the principles of health physics, persuasion is the health physicist's biggest and best tool. Effective persuasion requires effective communication. By effective

persuasion the health physicist should be able to accomplish his necessary work but he should always be
ready to insist and to stand firm to assure a safe
course of action should his persuasive efforts prove
to be ineffective.

Public communications in the health physics field
should be frequent. The bulk of the health physicist's
news should be good news. At all times, all levels
of communications should be truthful in concept and
detail, with careful precautions taken to guard against
omissions or unplanned distortions that may prevent
the true story from becoming known. To communicate effectively requires the stature to command adequate respect. A health physicist can command the
needed respect by repeatedly demonstrating his capability and good judgment to craftsmen, management,
and the public.

The organizational location of a health physics
program in a corporate structure is optional. Good
people will lead to a good program. In most situations an organizational position high in the corporate
structure will help to assure proper importance and
emphasis to the health physics program. In all cases
clear lines of authority should be established and
mutually understood by the health physicist, the
craftsmen, and management.

I. INTRODUCTION

The ability to communicate all levels of knowledge is one of man's unique abilities. To use this
ability to have good communications requires one to
think, talk, write and reason. The health physicist,
if he is to be effective in his profession, needs to
develop his communication capabilities with craftsmen, management, and the public. He can accomplish his necessary work only through effective thinking, talking, writing and reasoning.

He should devote sufficient time and interest to develop his skills in the field of communication and should assess from time to time his effectiveness in using these skills to accomplish his health physics assignments. A most important factor in developing good communications is the need to build confidence and trust between the communicator and the communicants.

II. TYPES OF COMMUNICATIONS

Communications in the health physics field may take all of the common forms. There will be day-to-day discussions and oral conversations. There will be written letters, notes, and memorandums. There will be well documented reports and publications, as well as detailed records for both technical and legal applications. In addition to these on-the-job communications, news to the public media may require the preparation of newspaper stories, television material, interviews, and meeting presentations.

A. To Craftsmen

Communications to craftsmen usually take the form of specific guidance in methods to accomplish their daily assignments. This may require the designation of work areas where radiation contamination levels require diligent attention. The establishment and use of time limits, protection equipment requirements, and work methods all require clear and persuasive communications.

One factor which is of prime importance, yet easily overlooked, is the technical level at which these

communications should take place. The health physicist should be sure that he develops the confidence of
the craftsmen through their repeated encounters with
his ideas and work. He should be sure to communicate with them using language, concepts, and terminology which are meaningful and understood by the
craftsmen. This does not mean that he talks down to
these people or feels superior to them, but merely
that he really communicates with them.

B. To Management

Communications to management provide an
opportunity to develop and advance the very best in
health physics programs. Again, the complete confidence of management is necessary if effective communications are to be provided. Close work with
management during the planning of new programs,
new construction, and all non-routine work can lead
to good health physics programs at a minimum of
cost. Good communications is an effective way to
keep health physics programs at economical levels.

Frequent and detailed discussions between health
physicists and management can be productive in defining the best ways to accomplish necessary programs
while meeting all radiological safety requirements.
The earning of mutual trust will greatly simplify difficulties during the discussions and planning part of
this work.

C. To the Record

A vital part of each health physicist's communications is the establishment and maintenance of good
records relating to the radiological aspects of the

work. It is necessary that wholly adequate but not
excessive records be maintained. The attention to
critical detail that may become vitally necessary when
the records are used at a later date for biological research or for legal actions should not be underesti-
mated. To provide intelligible and complete records
should be one of the major communication assignments of the health physics group.

D. To the Public

     Communications to the public are probably the
most misunderstood part of the health physicist's job.
Far too often it has become common practice to limit
public communications to the reporting of accidents
or near accidents. I would charge the health physicists with a new role in public communications. He
should be sure that most of the news the public hears
relating to radiological matters is good news. This
can be accomplished by frequently reporting successful completions of difficult tasks or continued successful routine operations involving radioactive material.
If and when an occasional mishap occurs, complete
and thorough disclosure to the public is necessary.
These communications should be made promptly and
accurately. There is no substitute for a precise and
truthful accident report. One needs to be on guard in
reporting accidental conditions to assure that misin-
terpretation or rephrasing of the report by the news
media will not distort or alter the truthfulness of the
reported accident.
     We all need additional skill in preparing news for
the public media and in expressing clearly the course
of events during interviews. An important part of

accomplishing public communications is the selection of terminology and descriptions so that they may be understood by the general public. This can become a difficult task but it is also a very vital task. It merits our best efforts.

III. METHODS

A. Gentle Persuasion

Second only to a thorough knowledge of the principles of health physics, persuasion is the health physicist's biggest and best tool. Effective persuasion requires effective communication. By effective persuasion the health physicist should be able to accomplish his necessary work. We all need to continually practice and develop our ability in persuading people to take voluntarily the proper action with regards to radiological problems. By building a good level of mutual trust and by demonstrating our capabilities at providing good balanced judgment statements we can effectively improve our persuasive position. Once craftsmen, management, and the public respects and trusts the health physicist, his job of communications and his job of completing health physics work safely is immensely simplified.

In spite of all his efforts, persuasion may not always be able to lead people to the proper course of action. When this is the case, the health physicist needs to insist on the right course of action and needs to assure himself that he is not overruled. We could conclude that he should be kind, gentle, and persuasive but carry the proverbial "big stick".

B. Routine Communications

Routine communications are very important.
They should be used to build confidence and to demonstrate the safety of the nuclear industry. As we said
before, most of the health physicist's news should be
good news. Routine communications should emphasize our ability to complete challenging radiological
work with a minimum of risk and extremely few
accidents.

IV. MANAGEMENT RELATIONS

A. Team Work

To accomplish radiological tasks a spirit of team
work needs to be developed at all levels of the organization. By pulling together to accomplish difficult
tasks and considering craftsmen, management, and
health physicists as a team, considerably more work
can be accomplished in a safer and more effective
manner. The health physicist can contribute substantially to the overall team effort by working con-
sciously to unite all working groups and to emphasize
the overall program and the value of the accomplishments to be obtained.

B. Organizational Considerations

The organizational location of the health physics
program within a corporate structure is optional.
Good people will make a good program, not organizational reporting lines of authority. Experience has
shown, however, that the task of the health physicist

is usually simplified if his organization has a rather
high position within the structure of components. It
seems to be a common practice to assign importance
and confidence to organizational levels as well as to
an individual's capabilities. Although good people can
earn the necessary confidence and function effectively
at any organizational level, the job is simplified if a
high organizational structure is initially assigned. A
high organizational structure emphasizes management's level of importance related to radiological
physics and radiological protection aspects of the work.

C. Balance Factors

Health physicists will earn respect of management by demonstrating good judgment and the ability
to balance safety, risk, and cost in the performance
of their assigned duties. Good management relations
should be established and maintained by all competent
health physicists. A substantial selling job may be
required when management fails to appreciate some
aspects of the radiation protection program but experience and good performance by the health physicist will undoubtedly prevail and favorable management relations will develop. It is particularly critical that health physicist's work closely with management in establishing general guide rules and policies
with respect to radiation protection. Neither management nor the health physicist alone should proclaim
such guides.

D. Authority

Lines of authority for various levels of action
need to be clearly defined and known by all. It is

extremely difficult and most unlikely that a good job can be completed when management and the health physicist are not clearly informed on their lines of authority.

V. SUMMARY

Lets be sure we communicate effectively and develop and use our persuasive abilities to accomplish our health physics work. We should assume a major role in developing a team effort on all programs involving any form of nuclear or atomic radiation. By using good judgment to balance risk, safety and cost we can earn the confidence of craftsmen, management and the public. Only through effective communications can we become effective health physicists.

Lets practive T^2WR—Think, Talk, Write and Reason.

PUBLIC RELATIONS CONSTRAINTS
ON HEALTH PHYSICS COMMUNICATIONS

W. F. Wegst
California Institute of Technology
Pasadena, California
And
G. W. Spangler
Chatanooga University
Chatanooga, Tennessee

INTRODUCTION

Public relations is a significant and important part of the practice of health physics. There
are many aspects to the relationship between public
relations and health physics, but this paper is
devoted to the examination of one which is not often
publicly discussed: The constraint placed on the communications of health physicists by the fear of adverse
public relations.

The discipline (or profession) of health physics
did not appear until perhaps 40-50 years after the
first use (or misuse) of ionizing radiations. Although
there were serious radiation safety efforts[1,2,3]

during this period, the publicity given the use of radiation was characteristically wildly optimistic and de-
void of any mention of possible danger. The public
readily accepted many radiation uses including diag-
nostic x-rays, x-ray treatments for removal of super-
fluous hair, general purpose radium and radon treatments, etc. As examples, note the following two
quotations: "The value of radium is unquestionably
established in chronic and subacute arthritis of all
kinds (luetic and tuberculous excepted); acute, subacute and chronic joint and muscular rheumatism
so-called); in gout, sciatica, neuralgia, polyneuritis,
lumbago, and the lancinating pains of tabes."[4]

"Radium has absolutely no toxic effects, it being
accepted as harmoniously by the human system as is
sunlight by the plant."[5]

This early gross misuse of radiation resulted in
many people being crippled and killed.[5] The misuse
was not due to a lack of basic information on the biological damage caused by radiation.[6, 7, 8, 9] The re-
quisite knowledge was available, but there was no
effective system for ensuring that it was taken into
account. There were profits to be made from the
sale of radiation services and equipment. Consequently
there was strong motivation for public relations which
emphasized the real and imaginary virtues of radiation. Thus, before the beginning of World War II, such
things as fluoroscopic shoe fitting machines were in
common use and much damage was done.

The profession of health physics was born as a
part of the atomic bomb project, [10] because the scien-
tists involved were concerned about the radiation
hazards associated with such a project. Fermi himself is said to have questioned the advisability of

proceeding with a project which would produce the radiological equivalent of tons of radium, [11] especially in view of the damage done by the approximately two pounds of radium then in use. Due to the nature of the project giving birth to the profession of health physics, there simply were no public relations problems. The entire project was shrouded in secrecy, in fact the very existence of the project was a secret.

The culmination of the Manhatten Project, at Hiroshima and Nagasaki, rather effectively eliminated the general secrecy surrounding the goals of the project and simultaneously engendered considerable public interest. Subsequently, the Smyth report[12] made the facts about the bomb and the hazards of radiation available to the public. While these events generated considerable public interest, real public concern seems to have developed after the 1954 H-bomb tests. The 15 megaton Bravo shot resulted in a major fallout incident in which a number of Marshal islanders, Japanese fishermen and U.S. servicemen were irradiated. Numerous radiation burns, several cases of radiation sickness, and one fatality resulted from this incident.[5,13]

By 1956, fallout and radiation hazards were a central issue in the presidential campaign. Since then, the 1957 fallout hearing before the Joint Committee on Atomic Energy, the Civil Defense Activity and publicity in the late 1950's, the Windscale reactor accident in England, the SL-I reactor accident, etc. have all contributed generally unfavorable publicity to the public out look toward radiation.

As the use of nuclear power and ionizing radiation find ever wider commercial use, public reaction to and public knowledge about radiation become extremely important.

NEED FOR PUBLIC RELATIONS

When the results of the atomic bomb project became public the need for a public information effort became immediately evident. The rapid development of nuclear reactors and other uses of radiation has made the need for a continuing public relations effort even more apparent. The Smyth report has been followed by a variety of public information documents ranging from the rather technical, "The Effects of Atomic Weapons",[14] to the elementary "understanding the atom" booklets.

This serious public relations effort has been necessary because:

1) Radiation uses and nuclear reactors are often associated in the public mind, with the atomic bomb.

2) A vast amount of publicity was given to radiation hazards in the 1956 presidential campaign.

3) Anti-bomb and anti-war publications have exaggerated or dramatized radiation hazards.

4) Special interest groups have tried to capitalize on radiation fears in order to block various atomic activities.

Clearly, efforts have been and are needed, to educate and reassure the public. The simple facts are:

1) Radiation is the best understood of environmental hazards.[15]

2) Radiation is probably the best regulated of all hazardous substances.

3) The safety record of the atomic industry is
   phenomenally good.

However, knowledge of these facts alone is not
sufficient to allay public fears. It is always easier
to make a dramatic, emotional cry of alarm, then it
is to reassure with generally dull and unemotional
facts or statistics.

PUBLIC RELATION CONSTRAINTS

The communication between health physicists and
the public, as well as intraprofessional communications have often been blocked for many reasons.
Government security restrictions constitute a
major constraint. Much work with radioactive materials is often associated in some way with a classified
project. The terms of the Atomic Energy Act are so
broad that many projects associated with atomic energy
can be considered classified.
Company proprietary restrictions often limit or
block effective communication. This type of constraint originates, obviously, from the desire of
corporations to maintain a competitive position in the
market place.
Economic constraints have probably had a significant impact on health physics communications. Operational health physicists often do not have time to write
for publication and they may only rarely be able to
attend national professional meetings. Local Health
Physics Chapters help in a limited way by providing
opportunities for informal communications. Nonetheless, the operational health physicist needs improved
opportunities for communicating with his colleagues.

Finally, the "public relations" constraints imposed by both commercial and non-commercial institutions often seriously limit the lines of communication in the area of health physics. The management of these institutions is often concerned with
adverse public reaction to the release of any information concerning work with or incidents involving
radioactive material.

Obviously, examples of the squelching or with-
holding of useful information due to public relation
constraints are difficult to document. Only rarely is
the public relations constraint as obvious as it became
at the 1964 annual meeting of the Health Physics
Society. An abstract of a paper reporting on the safety
problems connected with the operation of the SNAP-10A
reactor in space, had been accepted for presentation at the meeting. The abstract was published[15]
and several reporters as well as many health physicists had developed considerable interest in the paper.
However, prior to the meeting the paper was cancelled
and it was learned that the authors had been directed
to refrain from any discussion of its content!

In practice such situations are rare because the
public relations constraints are generally applied to
the abstract itself, only when a slip occurs do such
situations come to light. These public relation constraints and the need for numerous revisions and/or
deletion of material leads one to suspect that many
potentially useful papers are simply never written.
It is not uncommon to hear an experienced health
physicist comment that he no longer tries to get papers
through the obstacle course placed in the way of publication.

INCIDENTS UNREPORTED

The results of this situation appear obvious. A relatively small fraction of the radiation incidents, problems, and near-misses are reported in the literature. Of course, some incidents such as the Y-12[17] criticality accident or the SL-I[18] reactor accident are reported in great detail. On the other hand, practically any operational health physicist with a few years experience can recount a myriad of incidents and near incidents which were never published.

Most health physicists in Southern California know that a year or so ago, a contamination incident seriously limited the operations of a local firm. But what happened, how was the incident handled, how could it have been prevented, etc.? Very few health physicists can benefit from this incident, there has simply been no publication.

Another example of an apparent public relation constraint, concerns a serious incident of Co-60 irradiation in Mexico.[19] In fact, many health physicists probably do not know that an incident involving an inadequately controlled 5 Ci, Co-60 source, resulted in the death of 5 people in 5 months.[16] However, how did it happen, how can similar accidents be prevented, was the accident due to human failure or equipment failure? The open literature seems to contain no clues.

Finally, very few individuals know of the bizarre, but true case of an individual attempting to commit suicide by exposing himself to the beam of a low energy particle accelerator. Could such a possibility by guarded against, should interlocks be devised to prevent such an occurrence, what is done to handle a situation of this nature? Apparently, public relations constraints again prevented the free dissemination and open discussion of another near incident.

PROBLEMS CAUSED
BY COMMUNICATION BLOCKS

The lack of open literature on incidents and near incidents creates obvious problems. The operational health physicist cannot learn from the experiences of his contemporaries and must discover for himself the pitfalls and problems associated with each new operation within his facility.

While this situation is clearly inefficient and potentially even dangerous, the problem is even more complex. The absence of reports on problems and incidents causes difficulty in the relationship of the health physicist to his management. If, for example, there is no substantiating evidence to support the need for certain precautionary measures, the task of convincing management may be indeed formidable. The dearth of information about actual radiological problems (as opposed to hypothetically proposed problems) has the general undesirable effect of leading management personnel to the conclusion that radiological safety precautions are excessive.

HEALTH PHYSICISTS CAN
HELP IMPROVE THE SITUATION

Most organizations recognize the need for a public relations program, and few PR men are apt to like the idea of associating their organization with radiation and radioactive material, especially if people are involved in a radiation incident.

Although no fundamentally basic change in the system appears likely, the need for improved communications is manifest and health physicists can help to achieve this objective. The Health Physics Journal staff have expressed their interest in publishing operational health physics articles and notes.[20] Hence, publication is not a major problem. The principle requirement is to have sufficient fortitude and perseverance to get the papers to the publisher.

The first step is to decide if your experiences should be published, despite the difficulties. Then the question becomes—but how? Actually conditions vary so greatly between organizations that only rather general, broad suggestions can be made. With this in mind, the following set of ideas may help to placate your PR man and thus aid in clearing your paper for publication.

1) Know your public relations man. Each has his own concerns and areas of particular sensitivity. If you know what will be objectionable you can often find acceptable terminology.

2) Be positive; emphasize solutions and leave the reader to fill in the details of the problem. Discuss how good things are now, rather than how bad they were.

3) Avoid scare words; cancer, radiation sickness, radiation burns, leukemia, etc. are out. Say safety analysis, not hazard analysis. Take a tip from the medical profession, use medical

terms where possible (such as erythema or epilation). The phrase "deleterious consequences" can cover many unpleasant results, without hiding the causes and cures of a particular incident.

4) Generalize; the reader need not necessarily know that the incident took place in your facility.

5) Be mathematical; there are many ideas which can be expressed in mathematical form. Even simple summation expressions will quickly "turn off" most PR people.

6) Use technical terms and jargon. News reports are pitched at about a sixth grade level, therefore "hard words" quickly remove most any publication from the newsworth category. Few PR men will object to mention of high kerma or fluence, and few reporters will pick up on such terms.

7) Remember that management is usually not expert or fluent in radiation protection. Write your paper as if you were trying to convince your management of the need for a particular new program. Management may by inherently as nervous about radiation as is the public.

8) Get your radiation safety committee on your side. Radiation safety committees are made up of technical people who can usually be easily convinced of the need to disseminate information about radiation problems.

9) Keep trying.

10) As a last resort, get someone else to publish your paper, deleting all references to a particular organization.

CONCLUSION

Public relations considerations impose serious constraints on the free dissemination of information about radiation incidents and near incidents. However, health physicists can and should persistently work to overcome these constraints.

REFERENCES

1. R. L. Kathren, "Early X-Ray Protection in the United States", Health Physics, 8 pp. 503.

2. L. S. Taylor, "The International Commission on Radiological Protection", Health Physics, 1, 2, pp. 97.

3. L. S. Taylor, "Brief History of the National Committee on Radiological Protection (NCRP) covering the Period 1929-1946", Health Physics 1, 1, pp. 1.

4. W. B. Looney, Am. J. Roentgenol. Radium Therapy Nucl. Med. 72, 838 (1954).

5. J. Schubert, and R. E. Lapp, "Radiation: What It Is and How It Affects You", pp. 112, Viking Press, New York, (1957).

6. E. Thomson, "Some Notes on Roetgen Rays", Electrical Engineering, 22, pp. 520 (1896).

7. E. H. Grubbe, Radiology 21, 156 (1933).

8. J. Bergonie and L. Tribondean. Compt. Rend. 47, 400 (1904).

9. H. Heineke, Muench. Med. Woch Sch., No. 48 2089 (1903).

10. R. G. Hewlett and O. E. Anderson, The New World 1939/1946. (Pennsylvania State University Press, University Park, Pennsylvania, 1962).

11. "Lecture Notes: Health Physics Training Lectures, 1948-49", AECU-817 (1950).

12. H. D. Smyth, Atomic Energy for Military Purposes, (Princeton U. Press, Princeton, 1945).

13. R. A. Conrad, et. al., "Medical Survey of the People of Rongelap and Utirik Islands Nine and Ten Years After Exposure to Fallout Radiation", BNL-908 (1965).

14. S. Glasstone, The Effects of Atomic Weapons, (Government Printing Office, Washington, DC, 1950.)

15. The Biological Effects of Atomic Radiation, Summary Reports, (National Academy Of Science, National Research Council, Washington, DC, 1960.)

16. R. Alexander, and W. Sayer, "Hazard Analysis of Nuclear-Powered Space Systems", (Abstract) Health Physics 10, 8, pp. 624.

17. G. S. Hurst, Al., "Accidental Radiation Excursion at the Y-12 Plant", Health Physics 2, 2; see also AEC report Y-1234.

18. "SL-1 Accident", Atomic Energy Commission Investigation Board Report, June, 1961.

19. G. A. Andrews, "Mexican Co-60 Radiation Accident", Isotopes and Radiation, 1, 2, (Winter 1963-64).

20. "Request from the President to All Applied Health Physicists", Health Physics Society Newsletter, Nov. 1968, pg. 4.

MANAGEMENT REQUIREMENTS
ON HEALTH PHYSICS

Marlin E. Remley
Atomics International
Canoga Park, California

Most health physics and safety personnel occupy rather unique and very demanding positions in many organizations. Many of them feel they have large responsibilities with little authority and, hence, insufficient opportunity to discharge their responsibilities effectively. Others are alleged to have huge areas of authority with little responsibility for the results of their activities. These allegations frequently come through in adamant expressions as various operational activities are reviewed with personnel responsible for them.

Either of the above positions is a difficult and untenable one, and neither is representative of real situations. The requirements on the health physics and safety positions evolve from the demands on the managements of organizations. Thus, to understand the requirements on health physics and to develop effective response to managements' demands on their staffs, it is necessary to examine critically management responsibilities.

All managers are constantly faced with delivering some product—a working piece of hardware, a series of test results, a set of reports, or perhaps an effective expenditure of time on a series of research efforts—within a veritable host of boundary conditions. These latter usually include at least some of the following: A limited staff, considerably less than a generous budget, a demanding time schedule, stringent engineering specifications, and completion of the job safely. The manager's job is one of planning, organizing and implementing the plans to meet the above objectives while satisfying the boundary conditions. Since he needs help in a number of areas, he turns to strong support in a number of specialty staff functions; e.g., legal, accounting and financial control, public relations, and health physics. Various assignments are then made to these staffs, and the changes to the health physics staff can frequently take one or more of these forms: "Keep the operation safe, but don't interfere"; "We don't want any compromise in safety"; "No job will be done if it cannot be done safely." We are all well aware of these types of expressed attitudes toward the health and safety aspects of many jobs. With these approaches to a job, it is easy to see how the feeling of tremendous responsibility is developed by some health physicists, and further, how many people responsible for operations see the health physics staff as a bunch of obstructionists. But what do these charges really mean; what does management really want?

First, almost any manager recognizes that, if a health physics staff is to contribute effectively, some interference with the operation must be anticipated. It is axiomatic that, if the health physicist must work with the operational staff, review the operations, make constructive contributions to the operation, and then maintain some form of surveillance to assure that the health physics programs are implemented satisfactorily, he is going to perturb the operation to some extent. A manager would like this perturbation to be just that, as small a perturbation as the staff man can make it and still be effective in his job, and certainly not a major interference with program prosecution.

Then the health physics personnel should recognize that, in making his assignments, the manager is attempting to prosecute his programs effectively—not persecute his staff—and is depending on his health physics staff to tell him how the program can be implemented with acceptable risks. He is not interested in having his staff tell him that he cannot do something, but rather he wants to know how he can carry out the activities that need to be done. We are all well aware that advances in research and engineering development are the result of a continuing series of informed compromises, both technical and administrative. And usually, the effects of those compromises must be iterated into the programs one or more times in some form of systems analysis and review to achieve the most satisfactory set of results. Achievement of satisfactory health physics requirements on a program involves the same kind of approach and intelligent and informed compromise.

Thus, management needs a highly competent technical evaluation of the health physics questions in perspective with the operational goals and boundary conditions. This then will permit solutions to the problems, which can be effected without unduly

restricting the activities or adding unnecessary requirements. For example, it doesn't do one much
good to go out and purchase a fine color TV set if he
lives in an area where there are no color TV trans-
mitters.

Additionally, management needs a most critical
evaluation of the range of risks involved in his given
situation, not some hypothetical situation that the
safety man can conjure up. This evaluation must include the necessity for any safety factors and a judgment of how much of a safety factor it is prudent to
require in the actual situation under review. Too
large a safety factor or "cushion" will most certainly
result in no health physics or safety problems, but
may place unacceptable restrictions in some other
areas; i.e., the safety requirements may become too
expensive, or they may be unduly burdensome both in
time and effort. And sometimes the safety requirements hamper the operations while providing safety
assurances that are at best questionable. Thus a
knowledge of the manager's boundary conditions and
their ramifications must be included in the development of the optimum health physics and safety program.

Many "go--no go" situations are well described
in our regulatory standards. However, to provide
acceptable safety factors in many cases, most organizations develop internal company standards and criteria
that are somewhat more restrictive than those provided in the regulations. The differences in the two
sets of standards need to be clearly understood in
many applications.

It is incumbent on health physicists to develop
appropriate internal standards and criteria necessary
for the protection of personnel, to assure that the

operations staff and management understand the necessity for the standards, and then to administer them
judiciously. Further, the standards should be continuously reviewed, so that they can evolve as more
knowledge and information develop.

Both management and their health physics staffs
must be continuously aware of the subjectivity in many
of the evaluations of health physics questions and the
conclusions which the staffs finally present for implementation. Elaboration and improved definition of
this subjectivity are areas in which the health physics
staff can serve a most valuable role to their management. It is here that additional information and improved interpretation of the information in its application to the specific problem under study can contribute most effectively in management decision making.

The evaluation of the effectiveness and consequent
value of a health physics program is a source of continuing concern to management. As we are all aware,
outstanding programs together with excellent efforts
on the part of health physics and safety staffs usually
result in no adverse incidents; i.e., nothing unusual
happens. Hence, many valuable contributions to the
programs become accepted as more or less routine,
and there is a tendency to accept the program as
quite satisfactory without critical examination so long
as "nothing untoward continues to happen." However,
one should continuously be reviewing his health
physics program to assure that it satisfies his
manager's needs effectively, and not too redundantly,
and that it does not include unnecessary requirements
which go significantly beyond acceptable risk factors.
The manager must feel that he is getting value received for the portion of his organizations assets he

is investing in the health physics activities. I hasten
to point out that this takes careful review and evaluation to achieve the "happy medium" which should be
appropriate to an optimum health physics program.

It takes very few shortcomings in the way of poor
judgments and incomplete or improper analyses to
give pronounced negative results. Those which cul-
minate in incidents involving personnel injury and/or
major program delays frequently become evaluated
in highly subjective manners, and sometimes the
evaluations border on the emotional. In such cases
it usually appears to be much easier to assign values
to a poor program than to an excellent one. I guess
this must be accepted as one of the less desirable
aspects of being a member of a health and safety
activity.

Response to management demands requires
health physics personnel with more than just excellent
technical capability. Proper attitude, mature judgment, administrative capability, sense of responsibility, integrity, and character and personality to
project himself into the program requirements, while
providing the program evaluation from the health
physics standpoint, are all necessary for the health
physicist to be an effective staff consultant to his
management and to provide his management with the
appropriate expertise for management decisions involving health physics risks. The health physicist
must develop a real empathy with the operations personnel and maintain continuous communications and
understanding with them. The development of a sound
integrity throughout his activities is necessary to
achieve straightforward acceptance of his health
physics program by both management and operations.

In summary, the health physicist can meet the requirements of his management by carrying out the following in an effective manner:

1) Development of a program of radiological safety compatible with the operational activities.

2) Communication of his program throughout the organization at all levels. It is most important that personnel at the working level have a thorough understanding and acceptance of the program.

3) Continuous evolution of the program so that it can be continuously capable of satisfactory support to the operational efforts.

4) Continuing surveillance of operational activities to assure effective implementation of the program throughout all necessary areas of operations.

5) Continuing cognizance of the operational programs so that proper evaluation of health physics problems can be conducted promptly and made available early for the decision-making process by management.

6) Development of recommendations and approaches geared to helping his management meet their business goals and objectives with acceptable risks to personnel and investment.

7) Having the courage of his convictions if it becomes necessary to institute requirements which really involve significant interference in operational activities.

OPERATIONAL HEALTH PHYSICS—IN-HOUSE OR COMMERCIAL SERVICES

John S. Handloser
EG & G Santa Barbara Division
Goleta, California

Industry's use of radiation requires a large expense for health physics (HP) programs. In some organizations, including the national laboratories, large in-house health physics staffs perform essential HP research and development as well as the operational functions. Industrial users of radiation, however, require only the operational HP groups, a pure service function whose heavy cost is viewed as necessary overhead, to be borne out of profits. Although the results of this expense have been excellent—as verified by the safety record of the nuclear industry—I believe the time has come to critically analyze this cost to determine ways to reduce it. The health physicist is obligated to advise management on how to effect cost savings without sacrificing the quality of the HP program. Management should expect and heed these recommendations.

One method of cost reduction may be the judicious use of commercially available health physics services.

From those shown in the table, one can see that many
U.S. firms presently offer these services. This consideration will pose a fundamental question for management: Is it more economical to hire an in-house health
physics staff or use an outside commercial service or
consultant?

The purpose of this paper is not to make specific
recommendations to any given user of radiation. The
use of outside consultants or HP services can sometimes result in cost savings; however, many managers
prefer to establish complete in-house HP capabilities
after considering all factors. As we shall see, this
decision is merited, particularly in facilities that use
large amounts of radioactive materials.

Commercial Health Physics Services

Services	No. of Suppliers
Film Badges	15
Laundry (contaminated)	5
Leak Testing	30
Urinalysis	17
Radiation Monitoring	31
Air and Water Sampling	25
Waste Disposal	19
Instrument Calibration and Maintenance	29
Decontamination	22
Environmental Surveys	22

The reasons for NOT using commercial health physics services are as follows:

1. If the volume of HP work is very large it may be no more expensive to perform the task in-house than to purchase it from a commercial source. If the service is performed in-house, it can also be more closely controlled.

2. If the required service is too specialized, it may not be available commercially. An example is the specialized readout of film badges for particular situations. Brookhaven's problem of evaluating tracks from GeV particles cannot be solved economically by commercial sources.

3. There is relatively long response time to obtain results from commercial services. Although few facilities have personnel working close to the maximum permissible radiation limits, personnel monitoring and bioassay results for these individuals must be available quickly, in order to determine the work schedule for the next day or week.

4. The lack of quality in commercial services in the past has often deterred their use. (However, the commercial services have been improved as evidenced by the licensing of bioassay laboratories (discussed in this symposium), the various testing experiments and suggested standards for personnel dosimetry services, and the increase in the number of certified health physicists available for consulting.)

There are also many advantages to using commercial services, particularly for the small user, which may influence management's decision as to the practicality of establishing an in-house capability.

1. Commercial sources do a large volume of the same kind of service and should therefore do it better and cheaper. Personnel dosimetry firms, for example, process so many film badges that they can apply automatic methods of readout and recording and thus reduce the cost per reading over manual in-house systems.

2. A disinterested outside party performs the services. This has particular merit when obtaining data for environmental or personnel monitoring records. Records obtained and kept by reputable commercial services may be more acceptable in court than those from the organization itself, if the in-house operation is small and if nonprofessional personnel perform the HP tasks.

3. Purchased HP services are easily added to or cut back. As business increases or decreases, there is no necessity of hiring or laying off personnel; if new services are required because of a particular task, the services can be easily augmented.

After examining the available commercial services, the advantages of each, and his own situation the important question for the small user of radiation is whether he should hire a resident health physicist or use a professional consultant. If the necessary radiation protection problems require anything less than a full-time professional health physicist, I believe the manager should consider the services of a

consultant. If a health physicist is hired, his professional capabilities may not be fully utilized and management may find him doing technician's work at a
professional salary. Using a health physicist for
other technical tasks sometimes works, but it is
difficult to find the type of person who fills two positions well. It is also possible to train a staff industrial safety engineer to perform health physics tasks,
but this is usually expensive. The consultant specialist can perform the health physics tasks rapidly and
sometimes more economically because of his professional training and experience.

Commercially obtained personnel dosimetry
service has been reviewed extensively, and it is one
of the services to which costs can be assigned. These
costs have been calculated for my own organization
and projected to larger volumes of business. The results are given in Fig. 1. In constructing this curve,
I have considered beta-gamma film badges only, a
10-year depreciation period for the equipment, and
reasonable overhead and labor. It appears that we
must process a volume of between 300 and 500 badges
per month to justify an in-house capability. If our
load is less than 300, the costs are much greater if
we perform the services in-house rather than purchase them. Note that I believe the real in-house
costs never go below those of commercial services
even with the supplier's profit, because this profit is
more than offset by in-house overhead costs for
administration, record keeping, training of new personnel, etc.

The expense involved in establishing an in-house
calibration facility to repair, maintain, and calibrate
radiation detection instruments usually cannot be

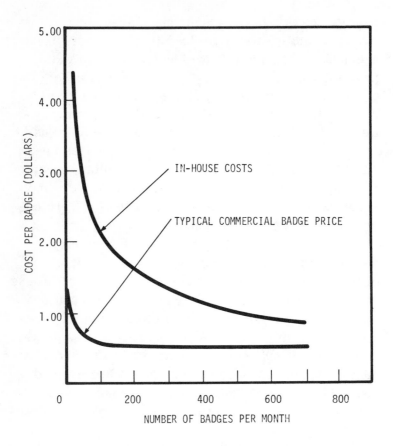

Fig. 1. Typical Film Badge Service Costs.

justified by the small user of radiation. Although offered by a number of commercial firms, these services are not being used extensively, perhaps because of the service time involved. Generally, extra instruments are required for use during the calibration period; however, the costs of this added instrumentation are usually small compared with setting up an in-house calibration facility. For example, an extensive standardized source setup or range is required to properly calibrate even a beta-gamma ionization chamber survey meter on all ranges.

Waste disposal and bioassays are usually obtained commercially for good reasons. Only the AEC and its laboratories, and some facilities with biological samples, dispose of their own radioactive waste. Most small users agree it is cheaper for a commercial source to perform this task. Bioassay determinations are so specialized, it is usually less expensive to employ a commercial service than to set up an in-house capability. Although certain well staffed and equipped biological research laboratories can perform bioassay services for their HP groups with very little additional expense. The usual user of radio-isotopes does not have this advantage.

In facilities with established health physics capabilities and instrumentation, infrequent gross activity environmental surveys can be performed with little additional expense. However, surveys for particular isotopes are more difficult and costly, and in organizations that lack the necessary equipment or available manpower, a commercial source for this service is attractive. Buying environmental surveys does not delay the health physics operation since the data are seldom required immediately.

In summary, the concept of buying health physics services should be re-examined by managers of health physics programs after carefully reviewing their individual needs. In new installations, setting up an in-house capability can be very expensive and unnecessary. In facilities with established health physics capabilities, phasing out these capabilities may be a subject for long range planning.

Personally, I believe the time is near when it will be common practice to contract out large complete

health physics programs to commercial HP firms.
Only a few such contracts have been let to date. To
the health physicist this should be a welcome idea because it would diversify his work. Managers should
also welcome the thought because it might reduce
their costs and relieve them of the responsibility of
the day-to-day operation of the health physics program.

MANAGEMENT AND HEALTH PHYSICS
INTERACTION IN A LARGE FEDERAL AGENCY

E. A. Belvin and G. F. Stone
Tennessee Valley Authority
Division of Health and Safety
Industrial and Radiological Hygiene Staff
Muscle Shoals, Alabama

ABSTRACT

This paper describes the unique interrelationships of Tennessee Valley Authority organizational
units which work together to control radiological
hazards in a variety of operations. TVA is a Federal
corporation created by the U. S. Congress as a re-
source development agency and governed by a 3-man
Board of Directors appointed by the President and
confirmed by the Senate. TVA's legislated responsibilities for controlling the Tennessee River and developing the Tennessee Valley are carried out through
program delegations to its several offices and divisions.
divisions.

The Industrial and Radiological Hygiene Staff
organizationally is a part of the Division of Health and

1683

Safety which must communicate with varying levels of
TVA management to ensure that potential radiation
hazards are recognized early in the design stages of
projects, that adequate controls are provided insofar
as possible before operations commence, and that
safe practices are followed after operations are in
progress. Within the Division of Health and Safety
itself, the professional health physics staff works
closely with medical, environmental engineering,
and safety staffs to formulate, implement, and keep
under surveillance effective radiological control
practices. The health physics program for the 3,456-
MWe Browns Ferry Nuclear Plant is used as an example of effective communications in designing and
planning the operations of a large nuclear power
facility.

INTRODUCTION

Before attempting to describe management-health
physics interaction in the Tennessee Valley Authority,
perhaps a brief description of the background, organization, and purposes of this agency might be helpful.
TVA was established May 18, 1933, as a corporate
agency of the Federal government in a physical setting
encompassing parts of seven states. The service area
is shown in Fig. 1. Its major policies, programs,
organization, and administrative relationships are
determined by a full-time 3-member Board of Directors. Members of the Board are appointed by the
President and confirmed by the Senate for 9-year
terms. The General Manager is TVA's principal
administrative officer and carries out programs,

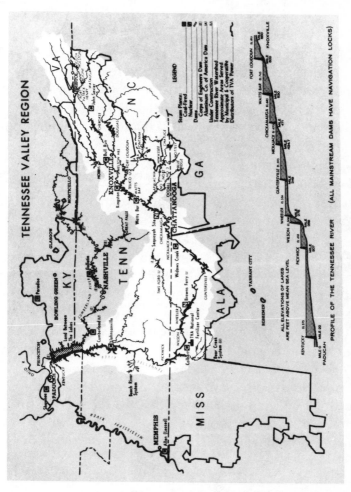

Figure 1.

policies, and decisions adopted by the Board.   Responsibilities for conducting programs, applying policies, and performing services are delegated by the Board through the General Manager to offices and divisions.   Figure 2 shows the general organization.

TVA's overall role is twofold: (1) To carry out the program of physical construction and operation involved in managing the Tennessee River to prevent floods, provide navigation, and produce power and (2) to work toward and provide the unifying influence and direction essential for the comprehensive development of all resources in the TVA region.   Major TVA programs include flood damage prevention, river navigation, construction activities, power production, fertilizer research and development, and tributary area development.

Use of radioactive materials and radiation-producing machines is expanding into a number of these program activities, and the need for management-health physics coordination is evident when one considers the diversity and remoteness of many of the field programs involved.   Discussion of all these activities is beyond the scope of this paper.   However, two program activities, construction and power production, require the fullest application of such close coordination, and means for effective communication and coordination of plans in these programs will be discussed in more detail.

COMMUNICATION METHODS IN TVA

TVA maintains a formal system of written administrative releases which define and communicate

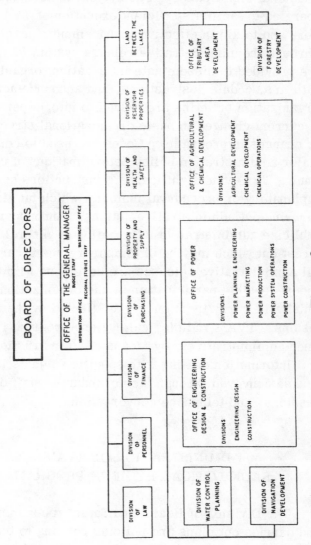

ORGANIZATION OF THE TENNESSEE VALLEY AUTHORITY
SEPTEMBER 14, 1967

BOARD OF DIRECTORS

OFFICE OF THE GENERAL MANAGER
INFORMATION OFFICE   BUDGET STAFF   WASHINGTON OFFICE
REGIONAL STUDIES STAFF

DIVISION OF LAW

DIVISION OF PERSONNEL

DIVISION OF FINANCE

DIVISION OF PURCHASING

DIVISION OF PROPERTY AND SUPPLY

DIVISION OF HEALTH AND SAFETY

DIVISION OF RESERVOIR PROPERTIES

LAND BETWEEN THE LAKES

OFFICE OF ENGINEERING DESIGN & CONSTRUCTION
DIVISIONS
ENGINEERING DESIGN
CONSTRUCTION

DIVISION OF WATER CONTROL PLANNING

DIVISION OF NAVIGATION DEVELOPMENT

OFFICE OF POWER
DIVISIONS
POWER PLANNING & ENGINEERING
POWER MARKETING
POWER PRODUCTION
POWER SYSTEM OPERATIONS
POWER CONSTRUCTION

OFFICE OF AGRICULTURAL & CHEMICAL DEVELOPMENT
DIVISIONS
AGRICULTURAL DEVELOPMENT
CHEMICAL DEVELOPMENT
CHEMICAL OPERATIONS

OFFICE OF TRIBUTARY AREA DEVELOPMENT

DIVISION OF FORESTRY DEVELOPMENT

Figure 2.

organization, policy, and procedural matters of inter-
divisional significance. The system is designed and
operated to facilitate efficient execution of TVA's
work and to aid in effective management control.
Through the administrative release system four means
are provided to disseminate information: organization
bulletins, codes, instructions, and announcements.
Organization bulletins are issued to inform personnel
of current changes in basic organizational structure
or changes in programs. Codes are used to convey
major administration policy determinations of continuing TVA-wide significance. Instructions contain
explanatory or procedural material which facilitates
carrying out administrative actions. Announcements
publicize administrative information of general interest but which may be of temporary significance.
All administrative releases are developed with the
widest feasible participation by the organizations
which will carry them out or be affected by their provisions. TVA's radiological hygiene program is outlined administratively by means of an instruction.

Information dealing with specific subjects is of
course conveyed through memorandums, staff discussions, and telephone conversations.

ADMINISTRATION OF TVA'S
RADIOLOGICAL HYGIENE PROGRAM

The Division of Health and Safety recommends
and carries out plans and policies relating to the health
and safety of employees and of the public affected by
TVA activities; to TVA's concern with environmental
sciences; and to the development and administration

of cooperative relations with other agencies in health, safety, and environmental science studies, demonstrations, and services. Figure 3 shows the organizational structure of this division.

The Industrial and Radiological Hygiene Staff of the Division of Health and Safety has principal responsibility for developing and maintaining a comprehensive radiological health program. For operations throughout TVA, it develops and describes standards and procedures consistent with regulatory programs of state and other Federal agencies including the Atomic Energy Commission; Federal Radiation Council; and Department of Health, Education, and Welfare. It reviews all designs and program plans involving radiation hazards and appraises each installation when radioactive material is used to assure conformance with developed standards. For TVA's nuclear power stations the staff will provide full-time onsite health physics services including personnel, plant, and environs monitoring. The chief of this staff is the Radiation Protection Officer for TVA. This provides a central point for administration of the radiological hygiene program.

A fully equipped radiological laboratory and counting room facility is operated by the Industrial and Radiological Hygiene Staff to provide radioanalytical services in support of all nuclear programs.

Personnel dosimetry and instrument calibration facilities are also operated to provide prompt and accurate determinations of employee exposure to radiation and to assure reliability of portable monitoring instruments used throughout TVA.

Within the Division of Health and Safety other supporting services for TVA's nuclear programs are

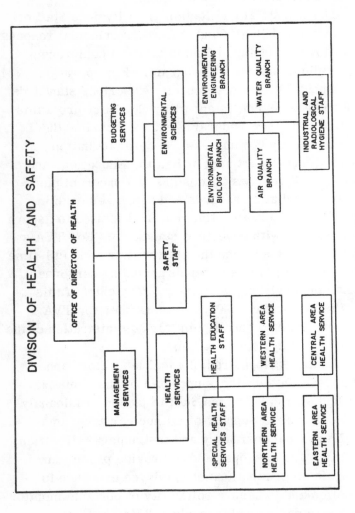

Figure 3.

provided in such related fields as employee health, environmental engineering, air and water quality, and industrial hygiene.

INTERRELATIONSHIPS OF TVA DIVISIONS AND STAFFS IN NUCLEAR FACILITY PLANNING

Coordination of several TVA divisions and staffs with the Industrial and Radiological Hygiene Staff is illustrated in Fig. 4. The Browns Ferry Nuclear Plant in TVA's nuclear power program is used as an example.

Divisional responsibilities were outlined very early in the planning stages of this plant, now under construction near Athens, Alabama. The Industrial and Radiological Hygiene Staff worked closely with all of these organizations.

The Division of Engineering Design, as a part of its overall design responsibility for the plant, developed specifications for engineering control of radiological hazards, including shielding, access control, and wastes management.

The Division of Water Control Planning developed integrated sampling and meteorological networks, including installing, testing, and calibrating field monitoring equipment; and, through its field staffs, services and maintains monitoring instruments.

The Division of Forestry Development praticipates in studies concerning potential effects of plant operations upon fish and other aquatic life. Samples of aquatic specimens are collected by the division and forwarded to the radiological hygiene laboratory for

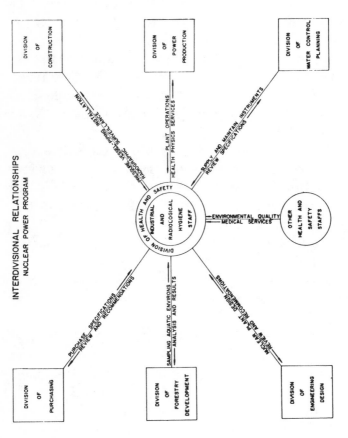

Figure 4.

analysis. This program has been initiated and will continue after plant operation begins.

The Division of Purchasing assisted in developing specifications for radiation detection instruments, laboratory assay equipment, sources, and other specialized equipment to be used in the radiological hygiene program.

The Division of Health and Safety played a significant role in selection and appraisal of sites which would meet requirements of the Atomic Energy Commission. Criteria pertaining to water quality and air quality, including meteorology and site dispersion factors, were developed and field background data were obtained. Complete review and analysis were made of the preliminary safety analysis report on all aspects pertaining to radiation and contamination control, particular attention being given to releases of radioactive wastes to the environment. An environmental monitoring program was established in collaboration with the Divisions of Water Control Planning, Forestry Development, and Purchasing. State and Federal agencies were contacted to assure adequacy and compatibility of programs. Inplant monitoring systems were designed and access control criteria were established in cooperation with the Divisions of Engineering Design and Power Production. Throughout construction there has been strict surveillance of radiographic operations conducted at the site by subcontractors. Radiological hygiene training was reviewed and schedules established with the Division of Power Production. Medical services and emergency plans, including intercommunication and assistance from other groups such as Oak Ridge National Laboratory and state health departments, were established.

Onsite health physics services for the Browns Ferry Nuclear Plant will be provided by the Division of Health and Safety. One professional health physicist and five health physics technicians will be stationed at the plant to provide continuous surveillance.

Another example of the interaction and coordination of several staffs is the radioactive fertilizer laboratory which was installed for research purposes at the National Fertilizer Development Center. Staffs in the Division of Health and Safety reviewed floor plans, operating techniques, ventilation patterns, waste disposal methods, and personnel access control. Recommendations were forwarded to the sponsoring division, and design changes were made to incorporate the suggested revisions. Assistance was also given in preparation of the application for a byproduct material license. Since operations began some 18 months ago, radiological hygiene surveillance has included radiation and contamination surveys, personnel monitoring, and bioassay analyses. The laboratory has been operated without any significant radiological incident.

SUMMARY

The radiological hygiene program for TVA is structured to fit a diversity of field operations spanning many division programs, some of which are remotely located. Thus, it is imperative that there be a very close interaction of health physics staff with management at several levels of administration. The program is unique in the fact that all programs involving work with radiation are coordinated early in

the planning stages through the Division of Health and
Safety and, more specifically, through the Industrial
and Radiological Hygiene Staff.   This staff reviews
each proposed operation for potential radiation haz
hazards and recommends approval or modification as
necessary.   The staff then works closely with the
sponsoring division to ensure that operations are conducted without undue risk to employees or to the public.   Effective planning and communications are
carried out in all TVA programs through administrative releases, documents of standards and procedures,
and memorandums.

A NATIONWIDE HEALTH PHYSICS PROGRAM FOR A LARGE INDUSTRIAL USER

Robert G. Wissink
3M Co.
St. Paul, Minn.

As a student graduating from one of the AEC Radiological Physics programs in 1958, I can recall that the list of potential employers included government laboratories, universities, public health agencies, and AEC contractors. There was little, if any, opportunity for an individual to consider private industry where radioactive materials were being used for their commercial value or as a part of manufacturing operations. During the last eleven years, I believe this situation has been changing and that with increased utilization of isotopes by industry there will be more demands for health physicists in this field. To support this belief I would like to quote a few figures. The number of AEC and agreement state licenses have increased by 65% over the last six years and Oak Ridge radioisotope sales increased 26.7% in one year alone. Both of these figures reflect not only the increased use of radioisotopes in the United States, but interest by new organizations which have

not used such materials before. An AEC employment
survey showed that in March of 1967, 429 private industries showed 35,457 employees in the atomic
energy field, an increase of 4.7% over 1966 figures.
During the same period, AEC contractor employee
figures at government owned establishments dropped
0.8%.

The 3M Company has been one of those organizations which has looked not only at the commercial
values of isotopes as potential products themselves,
but at how they can be used in research for new
product development and for quality control in manufacturing locations where older product lines have
long been established. As a result, 3M has been involved with quantities of radioactive materials ranging from 10 microcurie radium sources in static
measuring meters to 33,000 curie Strontium-90
sources used as heating units in SNAP-21 thermo-
electric generators. In between these two extremes
there are large numbers of beta gauges for quality
control, two research and development programs,
significant quantities of material used for a line of
commercially available radioisotope sources, and
until recently a specialized enriched uranium fuel
fabrication facility. With this amount of radioisotope
usage, one's natural reaction is to think the 3M has
a large health physics staff. Our situation is quite
the contrary and I wish to discuss it this afternoon.
I anticipate that what I have to offer will be of value
to those of you who are or may be involved in similar
situations in other companies.

Faced with the need for a staff health physicist,
3M Management decided in 1964 to place one in the
Medical Department. There were two main reasons

for this decision. The first, obviously, was that the
health physicist should be concerned with the health
of 3M employees. The second was that the Medical
Department functions across corporate divisional
lines. The position was established in such a way
that the 3M Health Physicist reports to the Manager
of Industrial Hygiene who in turn reports to the
Medical Director. The Medical Director reports to
the president of 3M Company.

During the last four years we have built a nationwide health physics program using the staff health
physicist and available personnel at our various plant
locations. This has been done by the establishment
of a radiation safety officer system where a Radiation
Safety Officer becomes basically responsible for the
use of ionizing radiation in his plant. Although the
R. S. O. organizationally reports to his usual supervisor, he has some additional direct responsibilities
within the R. S. O. system. These, of course, depend
upon what use is being made of radioisotopes. Right
now there are 31 R. S. O. 's in 3M locations around the
United States.

The R. S. O.'s have college or university degrees,
but with the exception of three people they have had
little, if any, previous experience with ionizing
radiation. In a typical manufacturing area, the
R. S. O. would be the plant engineer or the supervisor
in the quality control department. In our research
and development areas, the R. S. O.'s are radio-
chemists and these are the people with extensive experience in handling radioisotopes. None of the
R. S. O.'s are well qualified health physicists by virtue
of either training or experience.

To provide some similarity in background, all of the R. S. O.'s were brought to St. Paul in October of 1965 to hear 16 hours of lecture material during a two-day period. The lectures were given both by 3M staff members and outside people. As Table I shows, such topics as "Principles of Ionizing Radiation," the "Regulatory Program of the Atomic Energy Commission," "Fire Fighting Involving Radio active Materials," "Biological Effects of Radiation Exposures," and "Decontamination" were covered. Outside speakers included the Director, Region III Division of Compliance, a Health Physicist from the University of Minnesota, the Health Physicist from the Elk River Reactor, a Professor from the Univer sity of Michigan, and an official from the Minnesota Health Department. All of the lectures were repro- duced and bound into a manual which each R. S. O. could keep for future reference.

TABLE I

LECTURE SUBJECTS--R. S. O. TRAINING

    I. 3M Radiation Safety Organization.

   II. The Regulatory Program of the Atomic Energy Commission.

  III. State Registrations and Regulations.

  IV. Atomic Physics, Radioactivity, Half-Life.

    V. The Principles of Ionizing Radiation Protection.

  VI. Fire Fighting Involving Radioactive Material.

 VII. Laboratory Assay of Radioactive Materials.

VIII. Biological Effects of Radiation Exposure to Personnel and Public.

  IX. Industrial Uses of Radioactive Material.

   X. Contamination and Decontamination.

  XI. Effects of Radiation on Materials.

Although the training program was designed primarily for the Radiation Safety Officers, it was felt that the upper management group representing the various divisions from which the R. S. O.'s came should also be given some orientation with respect to ionizing radiation. Accordingly, a luncheon was held for them and the R. S. O.'s at which time a speaker discussed the use of ionizing radiation in industry.

We consider the formal training of the R. S. O.'s to be the backbone of our nationwide health physics program, but there are other facets of the system that make it work. The first of these has already been mentioned and that is the fact our Health Physicist's activities can cross company divisional lines. The second reason is probably equally important. In addition to being responsible for the usual health physics type activities, the Health Physicist also acts as 3M's Licensing Administrator for Radioactive Materials, and as Chairman of the 3M Isotope Committee. As a result, all licensing activities with the U. S. Atomic Energy Commission or agreement states are handled by him. This provides the Health Physicist an opportunity to evaluate the problems or hazards which might be encountered with each new proposed use of isotopes, to outline a radiation safety program suitable for the particular use, and to extablish an R. S. O. at the location of use, if one is not already there. Since 3M is composed of autonomous divisions, each source of radioactive material is licensed by division location. Both the name of the R. S. O. and Health Physicist appear on the license. While this means that 3M has a large number of individual licenses, it also means that each R. S. O. has specific responsibilities under his own license.

Some of the specific responsibilities of the R. S. O. are shown in Table II. The R. S. O. is to perform tests or measurements specified on the license, to assure compliance with applicable regulations, and to be continually aware how the sources of radioactivity are being used. He is to advise the Health Physicist of any unusual circumstances and arrange for periodic surveys. In some cases, the R. S. O. is directly involved in the handling of various types of sources, especially in research areas, and in these cases he is charged with keeping adequate inventories and doing his own survey work. He is also responsible for informing individuals working in and around sources about their potential hazards.

At the present time we have not extended the R. S. O. system to include other sources of ionizing radiation such as x-ray units, or electron accelerators. It is anticipated that this will be done in the future, and we are also giving serious consideration to expanding the practical aspects of radiation safety training by providing most R. S. O.'s with more source handling and radiation monitoring experience. The ultimate goal will be to bring all R. S. O.'s up to a point where they would be well qualified as health physics technicians. For the few that are already at this point, or beyond, we do not plan any future training, but will use them to help instruct others.

TABLE II
RADIATION OFFICER RESPONSIBILITIES

A. Perform tests stipulated on license.

B. Perform or arrange for radiation surveys.

C. Explain potential hazards of radiation to those working in and around sources.

D. Keep continually aware of all source locations and how material is being used.

E. Maintain records appropriate to license.

F. Assure compliance with 10CFR20 and 3M radiation protection program.

The use of radioactivity within 3M is going to continue to grow and we feel the R.S.O. system can grow with it. The number of R.S.O.'s is not limited and as the need arises we can add other Health Physicists to the Medical Staff to provide help for them. We had anticipated some relief from the need for specific licenses and R.S.O.'s in manufacturing areas due to the fact that many beta guages are now generally licensed units. However, our experience has been that this only makes it easier for a manufacturer or distributor to get the unit into the plant and that the restrictions on the user of a generally licensed item can create problems. There have been occasions when repairs have been necessary that could not have been done in a short time interval if we had not had a specific license and an R.S.O. As a result, we specifically license any major piece of equipment even though it might carry a general license number.

In summarizing my comments this afternoon, I think there are several important points. The first is that the type of system we have established is appealing to a profit oriented organization because it makes use of available manpower and does not add a large overhead staff. The second is that continuity throughout the country is provided because the program is centralized at the corporate staff level and responsibilities of the R.S.O. are clearly established

through the individual licensing arrangement; and
third, the training of R.S.O.'s can easily be expanded
upon as the need arises. There are, of course, many
details which I have not covered due to time limitations, but I would be happy to discuss them with you
during the course of the meetings today and tomorrow.

Session XI
REGULATIONS AND STANDARDS

Chairmen

DON C. FLECKENSTEIN
General Electric Co.
Schenectady, N.Y.

ALLEN BRODSKY
University of Pittsburgh
Pittsburgh, Penn.

THE IMPACT OF REGULATIONS, LICENSE CONDITIONS, AND INSPECTIONS ON THE OPERATIONAL RADIATION PROTECTION PROGRAM AT WASHINGTON STATE UNIVERSITY

Roger C. Brown
Nuclear Reactor Laboratory
Washington State University
Pullman, Washington

ABSTRACT

Washington State University has had a "broad" byproduct materials license for the past seven years. This license has been administered by the Atomic Energy Commission through 1966 and by the Washington State Department of Health since January 1, 1967. During this seven year period there have been many changes in regulations, license conditions, and five inspections by appropriate agencies.

The initial impact on the health physics group was that this maze of "red tape" and "harassment" by

1707

inspectors was of questionable value in our operational radiation protection program; however, subsequent experience has indicated that the impact of these regulations, license conditions, and inspections is one of the most desirable and beneficial aids to an effective operational radiation protection program for the following three reasons:

1. An outside agency passes judgment on the overall radiation protection program pointing out weak areas and implying corrective measures.

2. These agencies, along with their regulations and inspections, can effectively "request" the administration to implement practices and procedures which an operational health physics group would have great difficulty instituting.

3. The most important aspect is that by complying with these agencies to the fullest possible extent the maintenance of a high quality operational radiation protection program is virtually assured.

A brief summary of Washington State University's experience is included to illustrate the above three points.

INTRODUCTION

The administration and operation of a radiation protection program is a complex undertaking in any situation, but in a medium size university some unique complications arise. Prince[1] and Lambert[2] have described some of the organizational structures of the radiation protection group at various universities and the motivations behind these programs.

The organizational structure of Washington State University's radiation protection program does not differ greatly from their descriptions, and who can effectively argue against motivations such as, (1) protection of the health and welfare of personnel associated with ionizing radiation, (2) protection against future legal proceedings involving alleged over-exposure to ionizing radiation, and (3) to fulfill federal, state, and local regulations?

The primary purpose of this paper is to show in the following discussion that by emphasizing the third point instead of obtaining a lopsided program one will obtain a balanced program which will assure that all the above motivations are incorporated into the program.

DISCUSSION

Prior to 1960 Washington State University did not employ a full time health physicist, and the utilization of radioactive materials on campus was dependent, mainly, on individual specific licenses. With the advent of a research reactor and increased use of radioactive materials in teaching and research the necessity for the services of a full time health physicist became evident; therefore, late in 1960 a full time position of Health Physicist was filled.

One of the first tasks undertaken by the Health Physicist was to set up a formal radiation protection program and consolidate the many individual specific licenses for radioactive materials in one university-wide broad license. This was accomplished late in 1961. This license, in comparison with individual licenses, was filled with conditions, requirements, and references to regulations and previous correspondence.

Thus, it was not surprising in late 1962 after the first inspection conducted by the Atomic Energy Commission that items of noncompliance were noted by the inspector. Much like the "shake down" cruise of a new ship, difficulties in the operational radiation protection program were pointed out. Specifically, the items of noncompliance were for not leak testing sealed sources as required in conditions of the license. In addition the inspector commented on the lack of independent surveys of the various laboratories conducted by the health physics group and suggested that a system of surveys by this group should be instituted.

When these findings were made known to the University administration by the inspector at the termination of his inspection visit, the administration assured the inspector and the Health Physicist that steps would be taken to rectify the items of noncompliance and institute the inspector's recommendations.

The initial response of the health physics group was that this inspection was merely a form of harassment that interfered with the maintenance of a good radiation protection program. It was a wise member of the University administration, the late S. Town Stephenson, Dean of the Faculty, who set the proper course by requiring complete compliance with all regulations to the letter.

As a result of this first inspection two important decisions were made:

(1) sealed sources would be leak tested at six month intervals, and

(2) a graduate assistant to the Health Physicist was authorized to allow the health physics group to carry on an independent survey program.

Certainly the implementation of both of these decisions improved the quality of the radiation protection program.

From this point in time to the present the philosophy, if such a term is called for, of the operational radiation protection program at Washington State University has been to comply with all regulations and license conditions to the fullest possible extent. What have been the results of incorporating this philosophy?

RESULTS

Inspections

Since the first inspection of the broad license activities in 1962 there have been inspections by the Atomic Energy Commission inspectors in 1964, 1965, and 1966. Since Washington State became an agreement state in 1967 there have been inspections by representatives of the Washington State Department of Health in 1967 and 1968. In each of these inspections no items of noncompliance have been noted. Recommendations as a result of these inspections have always been given consideration and if possible put into practice.

Liason With Regulatory Agencies

Maintaining liason with the regulatory agencies is a worthwhile endeavor. If any question of interpretation of regulations, nature of regulations, or what agency has jurisdiction over a particular matter comes up, communications with personnel in the regulating agencies will in the majority of cases settle the issue before any mistakes are made.

Other Benefits

Another benefit, perhaps the most important, is the influence these regulatory agencies can bring to bear on matters pertaining to the expenditure of money on radiation safety practices. While the author is not aware of any published data on the cost of operating a radiation protection program in a university, Lenhard et al[3] have indicated that the health physics budget per employee at five research facilities maintained by Atomic Energy Commission contractors ranges from $45 to $265. In a university situation the cost figures are probably comparable if one can overcome the problem of differentiating between students and employees.

In any event most universities carefully weigh any request for additional funds in any area, and in the nonacademic area of operational health physics these requests are carefully scrutinized.

For example, take the case of the physics research project at Washington State University involving a study of the characteristics of the transuranic

elements incorporated into various crystal structures.
This project required working with 20-50 milligram
quantities of materials such as ^{147}Pm, ^{237}Np, ^{241}Am,
^{243}Am, and ^{244}Cm in an uncontained form. The
health physics group, at this time, had had no experience in working with hazardous alpha emitters of this
type and quantity.

Informal requests for additional personnel in the
health physics group to handle the additional health
physics work generated by this project were ignored
because the influence of the Health Physicist was not
great enough to outweigh other factions who considered
such a project routine.

This is where the matter stood when an amend-
ment to the University's broad license was requested.
Fortunately the Atomic Energy Commission recognized the hazards involved and requested further information before they would grant a license to possess
the material. This request for additional information was the deciding factor in convincing the University
administration to expend additional funds to provide
an adequate safety program for this transuranic research.

Thus, a regulatory agency's recognition of the
hazards involved in working with these transuranic
elements and insistence on adequate safeguards to
protect personnel and property resulted in measures
being taken to do so, which would not have been finan-
cially possible if the health physics group had to plead
its own case.

CONCLUSIONS

Washington State University decided to cooperate with the various regulatory agencies and comply with the regulations and license conditions to fullest possible extent in 1962. This policy has resulted in no items of noncompliance noted in five subsequent inspections by regulatory agency personnel; there has been a very effective and improved liason maintained with these regulatory agencies since that time; and in one very important instance insistence by regulatory agencies convinced the University to expend additional funds for radiation safety which the Health Physicist could not do with his limited influence.

In summary our policy of cooperation has these three results:

1. An outside agency passes judgment on the overall radiation protection program pointing out weak areas and implying corrective measures.

2. These agencies, along with their regulations and inspections, can effectively "request" the University administration to implement practices and procedures which an operational health physics group would have great difficulty instituting.

3. The most important aspect is that by complying with these agencies to the fullest possible extent the maintenance of a high quality operational radiation protection program is virtually assured.

REFERENCES

1. J. R. Prince, Health Phys. 9, 347 (1963).

2. J. P. Lambert, College and University Business 45, No. 3—78 (1968).

3. J. A. Lenhard, H. V. Heacker, R. L. Hervin, and W. T. Thornton, Health Phys. 13, 181 (1967).

THE IMPACT OF THE TRANSPORTATION REGULATIONS ON THE ROLE OF THE HEALTH PHYSICIST

Alfred W. Grella
Radiological Engineer
Office of Hazardous Materials
Department of Transportation

I am very pleased to have this opportunity and privilege to address the symposium today on a subject, which to a great many of you has possibly proven to be a source of some confusion—the regulations for the transportation of radioactive materials and their impact on the role of the health physicist. The last several years have been marked by very significant changes to these regulations. In particular the year past, 1968, represented a major milestone, insofar as the regulations of the United States are concerned, since, as many of you may be aware by now, a substantial revision of the regulations of the U. S. Department of Transportation (DOT) for transportation of radioactive materials was published in the Federal

Register on October 4, 1968. These amendments,
which just recently became effective, one month ago
today on December 31, 1968, to be exact, have now
brought the U.S. regulations into substantial conformance with the radioactive transport regulations of the
International Atomic Energy Agency (IAEA). Our
recent amendments probably represent the most far-
reaching, single regulatory effort to date by any
single nation in the field of hazardous materials transportation.

Much of the detail of the recent amendments has
been covered in papers at recent Health Physics
Society Symposia. One of these was presented at the
1967 meeting at Washington, D.C., and the second was
the subject of a refresher course at the recent Denver
meeting. I suggest these references as excellent
summaries of the new regulations. For this reason,
and also due to the limited time available to me today,
I shall not attempt to cover in detail all of the major
aspects of the recent regulatory changes.

My primary objective today, however, is to high-
light a few of the major features of the new transport
regulations as they relate to health physics principles,
and also to offer some of my own observations and
opinions on how these new regulations affect the operating health physicist might more effectively utilize and
interpret the regulations.

First, I shall review very briefly some of the
recent regulatory history. The responsibility for the
regulation of transportation of all forms of hazardous
materials is now vested within the DOT, under the
statutory authority of Title 18, U.S. Code, Sections
831-835. This authority rested previously with the
Interstate Commerce Commission (ICC) who, as many

of you know had for many years delegated most of its
authority, in regard to packaging of radioactive
materials, to the Bureau of Explosives, which is an
agency of the Association of American Railroads.
This authority was withdrawn in July 1966 by the
I.C.C. Subsequent to this, and concurrently with the
new cabinet-level DOT in April 1967, all regulatory
authority relating to shipment and transportation of
hazardous materials by all civil modes of transportation was then shifted to DOT.

Your author is presently employed as a health
physicist by the DOT, specifically in the Office of
Hazardous Materials, which is a staff-level office
under the Assistant Secretary for Research and Technology. Our office is responsible for coordination of
regulatory effort for all hazardous materials transport including radioactive materials between the four
modal operating administrations of DOT, i.e., the
Federal Aviation Administration (FAA) for air transport; the Federal Highway Administration (FHWA) for
highway transport; the Federal Railroad Administration (FRA) for rail transport; and the U.S. Coast
Guard (USCG) for water transport.

In my frequent daily contacts with other persons
in both industry and government, regarding the regulation of transport of radioactive materials, I have noted
that a substantial number of these contacts are with a
health physicist, or with some person who is in some
way connected with the health physics function within
his organization. I have also noticed that these persons' degree of familiarity with, and knowledge of the
radioactive transport regulations varies quite widely—
and in my opinion, is often disappointingly inadequate.
I cannot help but conclude that many health physicists

have, unintentionally perhaps, continued to prolong this deficiency for some time. The reasons for this may be many. Perhaps it is because the health physicist is not usually the person in his organization who is directly responsible for the transportation function, or perhaps it is because the nature of the regulations may, in the past, have made it diffucult to excerpt and locate those sections pertaining to radioactive materials, or perhaps it may be that many health physicists are just too often overly concerned with their radiation protection efforts within the controlled environment of their own plant, facility, or laboratory, without giving appreciable thought to the considerations which become so important once that the radioactive materials depart from this protected sphere and enter into the transportation environment, where they are subject to climatic exposure, rough handling during loading and unloading, vibration and impact, and accidents involving possibly severe effects, including fire—all while such radioactive materials are in the custody of transportation workers who are very likely quite unaware of any potential radiation or contamination hazards.

In any case, I hope that some of my remarks today will help a little towards clearing up any basic confusion that any of you might have on the regulations and point some of you in the right direction.

The basic consideration in the transportation of radioactive materials is that they may present radiation and contamination hazards to transportation workers, passengers, or the general public. In addition—and this has been the historic consideration—radiation exposure may damage other materials in transport—in particular, photographic film. Other considerations involve special problems, such as the potential for accidental criticality when fissile materials are involved, excessive thermal temperatures from decay heat of large sources, or on the other hand, more relaxed controls for less hazardous materials such as small or exempt quantities, manufactured articles or devices containing small sources, and low specific activity materials.

The newly developed transport regulation amendments, which are based on the regulations of the IAEA, accomplish the following, as summarized in Fig. 1.

MAJOR REGULATORY CHANGES

1.   More Emphasis on Accidents

2.   Reclassification

3.   Labeling

4.   Packaging

Figure 1.

1. More emphasis is placed upon the effects of serious transportation accidents on the performance of packaging.

2. A reclassification of radionuclides with associated packaging standards is now based on relative radiotoxicity considerations and the potential hazard of the contents, rather than solely on the type of radiation emanating from the package, as was the case for the previous regulations.

3. A new labeling system for radioactive materials, based on the IAEA system, is established.

4. Provisions are included for more types of specification packaging for radioactive materials, allowing more flexibility for the shipper, in terms of new package development, and clearer definition of the performance criteria which may now be used to evaluate the adequacy of new and existing packaging designs.

As a shipper of radioactive materials about to embark on his first usage of the new regulations, the three simple questions, as listed in Fig. 2, if initially

SHIPPER DETERMINES:

1. What Isotope?

2. How Much?

3. What Form

  a. Special Form

  b. Normal Form

Figure 2.

asked, will provide a logical approach toward more effectively and correctly using the new regulations:

1. What isotope is being shipped?

2. How much is being shipped?

3. In what form is the material?
    Is it in "Special form" or
    Is it in "Normal form".

In the determination of what the isotope is and
how much, the health physicist will often be called
upon, especially in the smaller organization, where
his sensitive counting and gamma, beta, or alpha
spectrometry equipment may be the only equipment
available, to provide such data, especially when shipments of waste radioactive materials are involved.

What do we mean by "Special Form" materials?
(See Fig. 3.) These are defined as ones, if released

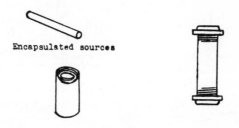

Encapsulated sources

Fig. 3. "Special Form" Materials.

from the package might present some direct radiation
hazard, but would present little hazard due to radiotoxicity and little possibility of contamination. This
might be the result of the inherent properties of the
material, such as its being in massive-solid form,
or acquired characteristics, such as an encapsulated
sealed source. The performance criteria which the
shipper must utilize to evaluate whether the material
qualifies as "special form" are provided in the regulations. Recognizing that these materials are much less
likely to get "scattered around" in the event of an

accident, and consequently less of a contamination
hazard, the regulations allow substantially larger
quantities to be transported, regardless of what particular "Transport group" the material would be classified if it were in "normal form."

　　"Normal Form" materials (see Fig. 4) are therefore defined as any materials which are not in "special

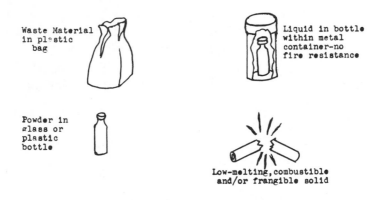

Waste Material in plastic bag

Liquid in bottle within metal container-no fire resistance

Powder in glass or plastic bottle

Low-melting, combustible and/or frangible solid

Fig. 4. "Normal Form" Materials.

form", and these are classified into either of seven
"transport groups", in a table of several hundred
radionuclides which is provided in the regulations.
Having answered the three aforementioned questions,
the shipper is now ready to consider the all-important
packaging requirements. The terminology "Type A
Packaging, Type B Packaging, Type A Quantity, and
Type B Quantity" are now introduced in the regulations.

　　The table in Fig. 5 indicates by transport group,
the Type A and Type B quantity limits. Note again the
importance of the "special form" determination, since
the quantity limits are independent of the transport
group. For the normal form materials, the increasing

TRANSPORT GROUP	TYPE A QUANTITY	TYPE B QUANTITY
	(curies)	(curies)
I	0.001	20
II	0.05	20
III	3	200
IV	20	200
V	20	5,000
VI and VII	1,000	50,000
SPECIAL FORM	20	5,000

Figure 5.

transport group numbers range from the more radio-toxic materials, such as the alpha emitters Pu-239, Am-241, Ra-226, etc which are Group I materials to the less radiotoxic higher number transport group materials, such as tritium in the form of gas, luminous paint, or adsorbed on a solid, which is a Group VII material.

Type A packaging (Fig. 6) is that which is de-signed in accordance with certain general packaging requirements as specified in the regulations, and which is adequate to prevent the loss or dispersal of its radioactive contents and to maintain its radiation shielding properties if the package is subjected to the Normal conditions of transport. The performance

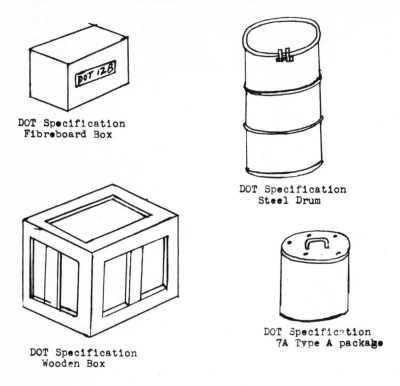

DOT Specification
Fibreboard Box

DOT Specification
Steel Drum

DOT Specification
Wooden Box

DOT Specification
7A Type A package

Fig. 6.   Type A Packaging.

tests to simulate these normal conditions are prescribed in the regulations.   In its development the
Type A quantity limits for Type A packaging, the
1959 recommendations of the ICRP Committee No. 2
were used by the IAEA as a basis.   Certain assumptions were made on the amount of dispersible materials which could be released (10^{-3} of the package contents) for an assumed accident severity.   Of this a-
mount released, a further assumption was made that
another fraction of this, (10^{-3}) or 10^{-6} of the package
contents would be taken up internally by any individual.
Then after a consideration of the uptake mode, i.e.,

soluble or insoluble material, by the general public and accident recovery worker, the permissible Type A package content for each radionuclide and uptake mode was then calculated. The radionuclides were then listed in order of decreasing radiotoxicity, and increasing quantity and placed into either of seven "transport groups", as shown in the previous slide.

The transport group and Type A package limits are also used as a basis for defining the package limits for small or "exempt" quantities, manufactured articles and radioactive devices, and for low specific activity materials. (See Fig. 7).

In the establishment of the Type A packaging limit for "Special Form" materials, an unshielded 20 curie source emitting 1 mev gamma photons, with a dose rate of about 1 R/hr at 10 feet was used as an assumed source standard. It was then assumed that a member of the general public might remain within 10 feet of a damaged Type A package for 3 hours (for a whole body dose of 3 rem) or that an accident re-covery worker would remain within 10 feet of the same damaged package for 12 hours (for a whole body dose of 12 rem).

Typically, Type A packaging includes those with which many of you are already familiar, such as the D.O.T. specification containers prescribed in the regulations, such as certain steel drums, wood boxes, fiberboard cartons, etc, plus a newly-included Speci-fication 7A, Type A general performance package. The intent of the new regulations is to prescribe the usage of Type A packaging within the framework of the packaging specifications provided in the regula-tions, without specific regulatory approval in the form of a D.O.T. Special Permit.

ALFRED W. GRELLA

TRANSPORT GROUP	SMALL OR EXEMPT QUANTITIES	MANUFACTURED ARTICLES AND RADIOACTIVE DEVICES MAXIMUM QUANTITIES		LOW SPECIFIC ACTIVITY MATERIALS
		PER DEVICE	PER PACKAGE	
I	0.01 mCi.	0.0001 Ci.	0.001 Ci.	0.0001 mCi/gram
II	0.1 mCi.	0.001 Ci.	0.05 Ci.	0.005 mCi/gram
III	1 mCi.	0.01 Ci.	3 Ci.	0.3 mCi/gram
IV	1 mCi.	0.05 Ci.	3 Ci.	0.3 mCi/gram
V	1 mCi	1 Ci.	1 Ci.	-------
VI	1 mCi.	1 Ci.	1 Ci.	-------
VII	25 Ci.	25 Ci.	200 Ci.	-------
SPECIAL FORM	1 mCi.	0.05 Ci.	20 Ci.	-------

Figure 7.

We shall now consider Type B packaging, (see Fig. 8) which involves packaging which must be designed to withstand, in addition to the normal conditions of transport, certain serious hypothetical

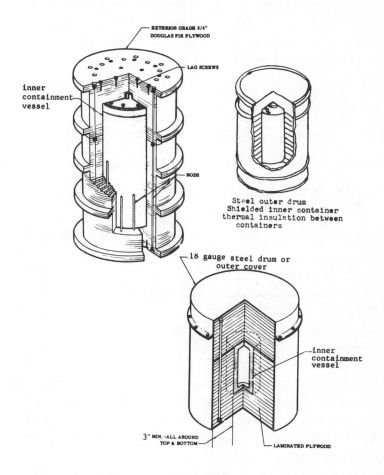

Fig. 8. Type B Packaging.

accident conditions with resultant limited loss of
shielding capability and essentially no loss of containment.   The direct exposure and uptake criteria as
were considered in the Type A packaging criteria are
not relevant in this case.   The performance criteria
to assess Type B packaging against hypothetical
accident conditions of transport are prescribed in the
regulations and include the following:

1. A 30 foot free drop onto an unyielding surface.

2. A puncture test which is a free drop over 40
    inches onto a six inch diameter steel pin.

3. Thermal exposure at 1475°F. for 30 minutes.

4. Water immersion for 8 hours (for fissile
    materials packaging only).

Except for a limited number of specification Type B
packagings prescribed in the regulations, all Type B
package designs require prior approval of the D.O.T.
under a special permit.   The continuing objective of
both D.O.T. and the industry, however, is to provide
in the regulations, as many specification package designs as possible, and continuing effort is being expended in this regard.

"Large quantities" are defined as those quantities
which involve greater than "Type B" quantities.   The
most common materials involved as large quantities
are the high-curie irradiator sources and irradiated
fuel materials.   Packaging requirements for large
sources involve all of the Type B requirements plus
other provisions for such things as decay heat dissipa-
tion, potential leakage of contaminated heat transfer
medium heavier shielding and the like, which in many

cases may involve a greater dependence upon administrative controls during transportation.

I shall not discuss the requirements for packaging
of fissile materials in any detail today, however, the
considerations for fissile materials are in addition to
those discussed previously. Again, as in the case of
Type B and large quantity packagings, except for
limited small quantities, and two specification packages
D.O.T. specifications 6L and 6M, which are available in the regulations, all fissile material packaging
designs require specific D.O.T. approval under a
special permit.

At this point it would be most appropriate to mention briefly the relationship of the regulations of the
U.S. Atomic Energy Commission, relative to transport of radioactive materials. In July 1966, Title 10
CFR Part 71, entitled, "Packaging of Radioactive
Materials for Transport," was published by the AEC
concurrently with a written memorandum of understanding between the ICC and AEC. This regulation
prescribed procedures and standards for approval by
the AEC of packaging designs for fissile materials
and large quantities of licensed materials and also
prescribes certain other requirements governing
such packaging and its delivery to a carrier for transport. Equivalent regulations applicable to the AEC
and its contractors are provided in the AEC Operating
Manual, Chapter 0529. In the new D.O.T. regulations, the interrelationships of these AEC regulations,
which are in addition to, and not a substitution for,
any of the D.O.T. regulations, are specified.

I would like now to cover two aspects of the regulations which might be considered as "operational"

requirements especially from the health physicist's standpoint. These involve radiation and contamination controls:

1. Control of Radiation During Transport—The new regulations, as well as the previous ones, prescribe that the maximum permissible dose rate at contact with the accessible exterior surface of any package of radioactive materials offered for transport shall not exceed 200 mR/hr, or 10 mR/hr at 3 feet (this latter value being equal to the maximum "Transport Index"). Higher dose rates are also prescribed, which are allowable provided that "sole use" of the transport vehicle is assured by the shipper. To control the radiation levels of accumulations of multiple numbers of packages once in the transportation environment, the regulations require that carriers shall maintain certain prescribed separation distances between radioactive materials packages and other areas which are continuously occupied by persons and/or photographic film. These separation distances relate the storage time against the "transport index," which was defined previously as the dose rate in mR/hr at 3 feet from the accessible exterior surface of the package. No package offered for transport may have a transport index exceeding 10. This "transport index" is also used as a basis for transport control of certain fissile materials packages, however, in these cases, the transport index value will have been calculated on a nuclear safety, rather than a radiation dose rate basis. The total transport index of any aggregate number of packages in a single transport vehicle or storage area may not exceed 50.

The new radioactive materials package labels, which substantially conform to those of the IAEA are illustrated in Fig. 9. To most of you these labels are a very significant departure in color and format from the old ICC "Class D poison" red or blue and white combination labels. The considerations for usage of these new labels, which are known as the Radioactive White-I, Radioactive Yellow-II, or Radioactive Yellow-III lebels, are summarized in Fig. 10. It should be noted that the new vehicle placarding requirement is keyed to the use of the Radioactive Yellow-III label, that is, on any packages for which this label is prescribed, it is required that the transport vehicle be placarded with the appropriate Radioactive Materials placard as prescribed in the regulations.

As a matter of historical development, the basis of the 200 mR/hr dose rate limit on the package surface may be of interest. This value which originated in the old ICC regulations back in 1947, was based upon a person carrying, in contact with his body, packages with the maximum permissible dose rate for 30 minutes/day. This results in an average daily exposure of 10 mrem, which although in compliance with 1947 standards, is in excess of more recent standards. Surveys in areas where a high volume of radioactive materials packages are handled and stored, have indicated, however, that current exposure standards are not being exceeded. Further study on this matter is also the objective of a recently undertaken effort by the DOT, AEC, and HEW on a Joint Survey of Radioactive Shipments.

The 10 mR/hr limit at one meter was chosen on the basis of "fast" film exposure limitations.

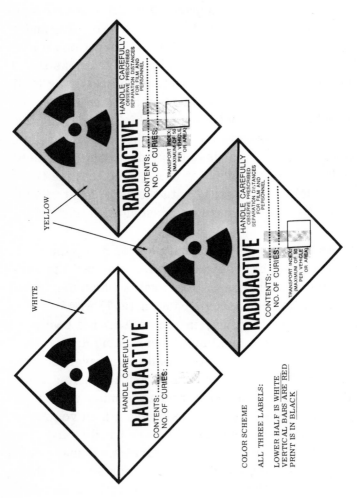

Figure 9.

| LABEL | DOSE RATE LIMITS | |
	AT ANY POINT ON ACCESSIBLE SURFACE OF PACKAGE	AT THREE FEET FROM ACCESSIBLE EXTERNAL SURFACE OF PACKAGE (TRANSPORT INDEX)
RADIOACTIVE WHITE-I	$\leq$ 0.5 mR/hr	0
RADIOACTIVE YELLOW-II	$\leq$ 10 mR/hr	$\leq$ 0.5 mR/hr
RADIOACTIVE YELLOW-III	$\leq$ 200 mR/hr	$\leq$ 10 mR/hr

Fig. 10.   Radiation Level Criteria for Use of New Labels.

2. Control of Contamination—The new regulations prescribe limits for non-fixed contamination on the external surfaces of packages and vehicles. A definition of the term "significant" removable contamination is provided and is listed in Fig. 11, along with the "significant" contamination limits. You will note that different limits are prescribed for uranium and thorium materials. The requirements for package and vehicle monitoring are no doubt much more likely to involve the Health Physicists activities directly than any other of the transport regulations requirements, since these monitoring requirements are usually always related to the Health Physics group in any organization.

Finally I would like to cover very briefly the sources of radioactive materials transport regulations. These are listed in Fig. 12. Of particular importance to any of you who are involved in export shipments are the IAEA regulations, published as Safety Series No. 6, 1967 edition. (See Fig. 13). The D.O.T. is the "competent authority" in the administration of the IAEA transport regulations in the U.S.A. I urge any of you who do export radioactive materials to become familiar with these regulations. They are extremely important.

Figure 14 lists the tariff sources of information on radioactive materials transportation regulations. These should not, as is done by many, be confused with the official regulations. They are merely publications by the originating agencies showing the acceptance and application of these regulations by the carriers concerned.

This completes my coverage of a few of the selected portions of the Regulations which I feel might

CONTAMINATION

"SIGNIFICANT" removable contamination is defined as the average amount, as measured in a wipe test, which exceeds the following limits:

FOR URANIUM (NATURAL OR DEPLETED) AND THORIUM

    Alpha   -- 10^{-11} Ci/cm^2 (2,200 d/m/100 cm^2)

    Beta gamma -- 10^{-10} Ci/cm^2 (22,000 d/m/100 cm^2)

FOR ALL OTHER CONTAMINANTS

    Alpha   -- 10^{-12} Ci/cm^2 (220 d/m/100 cm^2)

    Beta gamma -- 10^{-11} Ci/cm^2 (2,200 d/m/100 cm^2)

Figure 11.

SOURCES OF RADIOACTIVE MATERIALS TRANSPORT REGULATIONS

U.S.A. (as published in Code of Federal Regulations)

    1. Department of Transportation

        49 CFR Parts 170-189
        14 CFR Parts 103 (Federal Aviation Administration)
        46 CFR Part 146 (United States Coast Guard)

    2. U.S. Post Office

        39 CFR Parts 14 and 15
        U.S. Postal Guide, Parts 124 and 125

    3. U.S. Atomic Energy Commission

        10 CFR Part 71 "Packaging of Radioactive Material for Transport"

IAEA (International Atomic Energy Agency, Vienna)

    Safety Series No. 6 "Regulations for the Safe Transport of Radio-
    active Materials," 1967 Edition.

IATA (International Air Transport Association, Montreal, Canada)

    "IATA Regulations Relating to the Carriage of Restricted Articles
    by Air," Eleventh Edition, 1967.

Figure 12.

be of interest and importance to the health physicist.
It is on these portions that you are most apt to be
called upon for advice and assistance in assessing or
evaluating radioactive materials shipments. I urge
all of you who are not sufficiently familiar with the
new regulations, to make an effort to do so.

    I conclude by emphasizing that these new radio-
active materials transport regulations have been
established on basic health physics principles, and
now provide a degree of uniformity for all modes of
transport, as well as for international shipments.

SAFETY 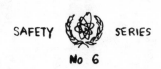 SERIES

No 6

Regulations for the Safe Transport of Radioactive Materials

1967 Edition

INTERNATIONAL ATOMIC ENERGY AGENCY

VIENNA 1967

Fig. 13.   IAEA Regulations.

Agent T. C. George's Tariff No. 19, publishing the "Department of Transportation Regulations for Transportation of Explosives and Other Dangerous Articles by Land and Water and in Rail Freight Service and by Motor Vehicle (Highway), Water Including Specifications for Shipping Containers." Available from: Bureau of Explosives, AAR, 2 Pennsylvania Plaza, New York, New York 10001.

Motor Carriers Explosives and Dangerous Articles Tariff, "Dangerous Articles Tariff No. 13," September, 1967. Published by and available from: American Trucking Associations, Inc., 1616 P Street, N.W., Washington, D. C.

"Official Air Transport Restricted Articles Tariff No. 6-D," governing the transportation of restricted articles by air. Published by and available from: Airline Publishers, Inc., Agent, Washington, D. C.

Fig. 14. Official Tariff Publications Which Include Regulations for Radioactive Materials Transportation.

The major impact on the role of the operating health physicist is that he has no less responsibility to educate himself on these regulations as he does on any of the other radiation protection standards.

REFERENCES

1. Code of Federal Regulations, Title 49 Parts 171-178, plus amendments thereto, Vol. 33, Number 194, October 4, 1968.

2. Safety Series No. 6, Regulations for the Safe Transport of Radioactive Materials, 1967 Edition, IAEA, Vienna.

3. R. Gibson (Editor), The Safe Transport of Radioactive Materials, Pergamon Press, 1966.

4. W. A. Brobst, "The New Look in Transportation Regulations", Health Physics Society Meeting, Washington, D. C., June 22, 1967.

5. P. Colsmann, "Transportation Regulations for Radioactive Materials", Health Physics Society Meeting, Denver, Colorado, June 20, 1968.

6. R. W. Blackburn, "The Transportation of Radioactive Materials", Canadian Nuclear Association Conference, May 1967, Montreal, Quebec.

THE PRINCIPLES OF DERIVED WORKING LIMITS AND INVESTIGATION LEVELS IN RATIONALISING THE DESIGN AND INTERPRETATION OF MONITORING PROGRAMMES

H. J. Dunster* and T. F. Johns**

INTRODUCTION

Monitoring is an ill-defined term which has come to mean little more than the taking of measurements associated with radiological protection. It is better regarded as a complex and sophisticated process involving not merely the taking of measurements but also their interpretation. The principal objectives of monitoring are to help to achieve safety and also

*Radiological Protection Division, UKAEA Health and Safety Branch, Harwell, Didcot, Berks., England.
**Radiological and Safety Division, Atomic Energy Establishment, Winfrith, Dorchester, Dorset, England.

to demonstrate that safety has been satisfactorily achieved. It may be intended to detect changes in working conditions, or to demonstrate compliance with radiation standards, or, and this is true in the majority of cases, both. In any event, no monitoring measurement can be said to be appropriate unless, either alone or in combination with others, it can be used as the basis for a decision or a conclusion bearing on safety. Monitoring is a tool, a technique, of radiological protection, it is not an end in itself.

This paper is concerned with monitoring aimed at achieving or demonstrating the safety of the individual. It is not concerned with monitoring solely aimed at detecting plant abnormalities, important though this problem is.

The basic standards of radiological protection are those recommended by the International Commission on Radiological Protection, with which almost all national standards are broadly compatible. Unfortunately, few monitoring measurements show results which are directly expressible in ICRP terms. In some cases, interpretation in these terms is easy if simplifying assumptions are made. For example, the results of individual monitoring for external radiation can be interpreted by taking the measured dose from penetrating radiation as directly equal to that received by the internal organs of the body and the measured dose from total radiation as that received by the skin. In other cases, there can be no such simple link between the measurement and the basic standard because the interpretation of the measurement depends, for example, on the past, present and future behaviour of the individuals within their environment. Not surprisingly, there is now considerable

diversity in the methods of using measurements of
this kind in a radiological protection programme. It is
the aim of this paper to show how the use of two simple concepts, the derived working limit and the investigation level, can be used to rationalise both the
design and interpretation of radiological monitoring
programs.

THE CONCEPT OF THE
DERIVED WORKING LIMIT

Perhaps the most obvious way of using the results of monitoring measurements, where these
cannot be expressed directly in terms of the radiation standards, is to use the results, either individ-
ually or in combination, to calculate doses or other
quantities for which basic standards do exist. This
method is clearly the method of choice when such calculations are simple. It is the usual method for interpreting the results of individual monitoring for
external radiation and for making use of dose-rate
measurements preceding an operation of limited
duration for which an acceptable dose can be defined.
However, for many forms of monitoring, especially for monitoring in the working or public environment, it is easier to work from the basic standards backwards and to establish a figure, closely
related to the practical measurement, which is derived from the basic standard. This secondary stand
ard can then be called a derived working limit. The
value adopted will be dependent on the assumptions
made in the calculations, that is, on the model select

for relating the basic standard to the measurement.
The accuracy of the derived working limit will depend principally on how closely this model represents the true situation on any single occasion.   The
choice of model will in any case be a compromise.
On the one hand, a highly generalised model will give
a DWL which will be widely applicable but which will,
in any particular situation, not accurately reflect
the basic standard from which it is derived.   In order
to ensure safety, the model will have to be selected
conservatively so that in most cases the DWL will
contain a safety factor, often a substantial safety
factor.   On the other hand, the model can be chosen
to be highly specific and thus to represent closely
the situation it is intended to reflect.   It will then
accurately reflect the basic standard in the circumstances for which it is designed, but will be inappro-
priate in all other circumstances.   Two examples in
common use show the extremes of this situation.

Almost all countries and institutions make use
of surface contamination monitoring and have established limiting or permissible values for these
measurements which are losely related to the maximum permissible doses and intakes of ICRP.   The
relationship between surface contamination and these
quantities is extremely tenuous and depends critically
on many operational and environmental factors.   All
that can be reliably said of the DWL in this case is
that compliance with it provides a high degree of
assurance that the general standards of housekeeping
are such that intakes by inhalation and external radiation doses from the surface contamination itself will
both be below the ICRP recommendations.   At the
other extreme is the establishment of a DWL of

discharges of radioactive waste to a river used for
drinking water. In this case, provided that the problem is not too severely complicated by, for example,
sedimentation, a close relationship can be established
between the discharge and the dose to the consumers
of the river water. The DWL then reflects the basic
standard with considerable accuracy. Even here,
however, it will still contain some margin for uncertainty, perhaps for years of abnormally low river
flow. It is thus generally true that a DWL will be
more conservative than the basic standards which
underly it. Compliance with the DWL will then indicate that the basic standards are complied with but
will not necessarily provide a numerical indication of
the margin of safety.

The presence of this margin of safety and particularly its variability in different conditions means
that derived working limits must be applied with care
and common sense. Thus, the DWL for surface contamination can usefully be incorporated into management instructions or even into regulations, provided
that there is adequate recognition that circumstances
alter cases. All too often, however, this recognition
is lacking.

While it is clear that the use of derived working
limits rationalises the interpretation of monitoring
programmes, their impact on design is more indirect
and less obvious. In practice, however, the collection
of the information needed to establish a DWL gives
an insight into the way in which the different types of
monitoring available relate to the basic standards, and
this insight contributes substantially to the choice of
monitoring methods and to the inter-relationship between different forms of monitoring. Thus, a study of

derived working levels in foodstuffs in an environmental investigation will pinpoint the critical pathways, the critical nuclides and the critical population, and can convert an ill-designed programme in which samples are taken almost at random into a much more valuable and almost always cheaper programme, in which a limited number of environmental materials are sampled on a logical basis and analysed for the materials of greatest importance. Subsequently, a comparison of the results obtained with the derived working limits may well indicate that some parts of the programme are of trivial value and can be reduced or abandoned as experience is gained. It is always difficult to reduce a monitoring programme because the process savours of lowering the standards of safety. The derived working limit provides a useful objective standard for taking these difficult decisions.

THE CONCEPT OF INVESTIGATION LEVELS

A great deal of monitoring is of a confirmatory nature. Experience, often over many years, indicates that working conditions are satisfactory, but some confirmation of this is needed and is provided by a monitoring programme. Only if the results of this programme are unusual or unsatisfactory is any action called for. For example, much monitoring of radiation dose rates in workplaces and of surface contamination is done by observing a meter reading at a large number of locations, but recording the results only when the meter readings are of special interest. This process requires the introduction, either implicitly or explicitly, of an investigation level which can be defined as the numerical value of a reading above which the result is sufficiently important to justify further investigations or enquiries, such as a review of the circumstances causing it or an assessment of the consequences.

The primary value of the concept of an investigation level is that it reduces the effort employed in interpreting, or indeed even recording, trivial information and allows more attention to be paid to results which are of genuine significance. In many cases, as in the two examples quoted above, it allows substantially more thorough monitoring to be carried out than would otherwise be possible. Another advantage of the concept is that it allows remedial action to be taken progressively. When an investigation level is exceeded, questions are asked and recommendations for improvement may follow. Often, however, these investigations will show that the situation was transient and unimportant and no further action is called for. Operations may then be continued, even though investigation levels may be frequently exceeded, without this representing a hazardous situation. There will, however, be a commitment of effort needed to conduct the investigations and this will encourage remedial action. In more extreme cases, the DWL will be exceeded and even if this does not necessarily imply an infringement of the basic standards it does represent a departure from the working standards adopted by management and is thus a positive indication of the need for remedial measures. In applying this progression, it is important to remember that an investigation level will normally apply to a single result whereas a derived working limit usually applies to

the average or total over a period which, in the case
of some environmental limits, may be as long as a
year.

One of the best examples of an investigation level
is that used in ICRP Publication 10[2] for deciding when
to proceed with a detailed interpretation of a measurement of internal bodily contamination. In this field,
the interpretation is often more complex than the
measurement and it is of considerable importance
not to waste effort in interpreting trivial situations
too precisely. The basic investigation level adopted
in ICRP Publication 10 is the intake to the body of
1/10 of the permissible quarterly intake, i.e. 1/20 of
the permissible annual intake. This basic investigation level is then converted on the basis of suitable
metabolic models to derived investigation levels
(DIL) for the amounts excreted in urine and the a-
mounts retained in the body. The DIL is a function
of the time after a single intake equal to the investigation level. When the time and number of intakes is
unknown, it may conservatively be assumed that all
the intakes took place immediately after the previous
monitoring measurement. With this interpretation,
if the results of a programme of individual monitoring,
either of excreta or of whole body measurements, are
all below the relevant values of DIL, then it is quite
certain that the total intake in any period between
monitoring measurements has not exceeded the investigation level. Since the investigation level is only
1/20 of the permissible annual intake, this also gives
assurance that the total annual intake is well below
the permissible value.

This use of investigation levels has its most obvious impact on the interpretation of monitoring

programmes, but can also be used in simplifying their
design. In particular, a combination of the values of
derived investigation levels as a function of time and
of the available sensitivity of monitoring methods
gives good guidance of the maximum interval that can
be allowed between successive determinations. Con-
versely, if the interval is fixed by other considerations, such as the variability of the work in progress,
then the derived investigation level gives an indication of the sensitivity needed and may thus allow
economies to be made in analytical or measurement
techniques.

In the monitoring of external radiation, it is
usually cheaper, more satisfactory and more convenient to monitor individuals rather than to monitor
their environment. As a result, many individuals
carry monitoring devices, even though the radiation
doses they receive are trivial by comparison with
the maximum permissible doses. For several·years
now, ICRP recommendations have made it clear that
these low doses need not be established by individual
monitoring. The results can therefore be regarded
as providing a general confirmation of satisfactory
conditions rather than forming an individual dose
record. However, it has in practice become conventional to note and record all radiation doses above the
threshold of detection of the personal dosemeter.
Other exposures, often of the same order of magnitude,
are not recorded, either because they are below the
threshold of detection or because individuals are not
monitored. The original intention of ICRP would be
met by establishing an investigation level based on
logical grounds and not merely on the sensitivity of
detection, below which the doses could be disregarded

and not recorded. The investigation level would have
to be chosen sufficiently low for the neglect of data at
low levels to have no significant effect either on the
value of the personal dose records or on the control
of the situation in workplaces. ICRP has now recommended that the investigation level for penetrating
radiation should be set at 50 mrem for a dosemeter
issued for 2 weeks, 100 mrem for 1 month, 300 mrem
for 3 months.[3] Annual doses accumulated at levels
below the investigation level would then always be less
than 3/10 of the maximum permissible annual dose,
the figure for which the Commission requires individual monitoring and personal records.

  With the present widespread issue of personal
dosemeters, the adoption of these investigation levels
would mean that the great majority of workers would
have a radiation dose record which merely identified
them and stated that their doses had always been
below these investigation levels. Some technical
simplifications would follow from the removal of the
need to measure very low doses, but the main benefits would be a greatly simplified personal record
system. In the absence of such simplification, the
increased use of radiation sources and the movement
of employees between employers and between countries
will result in a complexity of record keeping which is
totally out of proportion to the hazards, if any, of
these low doses of radiation.

GENERAL CONCLUSIONS

  The combined use of derived working limits and
investigation levels with a clear understanding of the

distinction between them can lead to a rationalising and a simplifying of the interpretation of monitoring programmes. This in itself is beneficial because it helps to prevent such programmes from sinking into meaningless repetition. The derived working levels allow conclusions to be drawn routinely and without difficulty from the monitoring results, while the investigation levels focus attention on the significant results and show where improvements are most likely to be needed. They both provide standards of comparison which can be used in the revision of the monitoring programme as experience develops.

If a monitoring programme produces results for which neither derived working limits nor investigation levels have been set, there should be an onus on the health physicist to show reason why his programme should not be withdrawn and his funds and staff reduced accordingly.

REFERENCES

1. Recommendations of the International Commission on Radiological Protection (Adopted September 17, 1965). ICRP Publication 9, Pergamon Press, Oxford (1966).

2. Evaluation of Radiation Doses to Body Tissues from Internal Contamination due to Occupational Exposure: A Report by Committee 4 of the International Commission on Radiological Protection. ICRP Publication 10, Pergamon Press, Oxford (1968).

3. General Principles of Monitoring for Radiation Protection of Workers: A Report by Committee 4 of the International Commission on Radiological Protection. ICRP Publication 12, Pergamon Press, Oxford (1969).

CRITICALITY DETECTION SYSTEM—A PLEA
FOR CURRENT CRITERIA

D. H. Denham and J. M. Selby
Battelle Memorial Institute
Pacific Northwest Laboratory
Richland, Washington

ABSTRACT

Comparison of existing criticality detection system criteria and regulations to criteria and regulations for other phases of the nuclear industry is rather
startling. USASI has developed a standard on an
evacuation signal but has not developed a standard on
a criticality detection system. The regulatory organization of the AEC requires, in 10 CFR 70, the use of
criticality detectors but provides little guidance on
the requirements for such a system. The guidance
provided in AEC Manual Chapters for AEC contractors is even less than that for the licensee. Several
papers on criticality accidents, which have been reported in the Health Physics Journal, mention the
role that criticality detectors played in alerting

personnel. However, none of these contain recommendations for such a system.

The existing standards for criticality detection systems and the regulations governing their use are discussed. The evolution of a fail-safe neutron criticality alarm system at Battelle-Northwest, with capabilities that surpass the existing regulations, is described. New standards which have been proposed will provide better guidance for criticality detection systems. Results of tests of the system's components are compared to illustrate the practicability of meeting the new proposed standards.

INTRODUCTION

With the growth of the nuclear industry, personnel protection methods and programs have become more sophisticated technically, more standardized in practice and generally more covered by codes and regulations. These requirements for sophistication are evident when reviewing as many as 50 handbooks, reports, codes or regulations, which an employer may find useful or applicable in establishing a radiation protection program suitable to his needs. However, there is at least one phase of the radiation protection program, the criticality detection and alarm system, which has been neglected seriously in the regulations and handbooks.

Mr. K. J. Aspinall in his article, "Criticality Detection and Alarm Systems", stated, "A criticality alarm system is a rescue device. It is evoked when prevention has failed.—It is a last ditch defense designed to operate when all else has failed." Be honest with yourself, will your criticality detection and alarm system operate when all else has failed? Will your personnel respond immediately if it sounds or have they been subjected to too many false alarms?

PRESENT STANDARDS AND REGULATIONS

One might assume that adherence to the established codes and regulations would place you in a position that your criticality alarm system will work when all else has failed, as suggested by Mr. Aspinall. Reviewing the Code of Federal Regulations, Title 10, Section 70.24, it is noted that a requirement exists for a "monitoring system, including gamma or neutron-sensitive radiation devices which will energize clearly audible alarm signals in the event a condition of criticality occurs which generates radiation levels of 300 rem per hour one foot from the source." It is further stated that the alarm point of the device shall be set not less than 5 mrem per hour and not more than 20 mrem per hour. The final requirement restricts the distance between the detector and source to 120 feet or less depending on the intervening shielding.

AEC Manual Chapter Appendix 8401 provides even less guidance in stating "Physical controls should act to preclude criticality except under very deliberate and carefully controlled circumstances and should assure that automatic alarms and countermeasures will be initiated in the event inadvertent criticality or excessive radiation levels are achieved."

The USASI Standards include one, N2.3, "Immediate Evacuation Signal", which contains 12 pages of description on what is required technically to provide a unique audible signal and what testing procedure should be followed to assure proper operation. However, there is no USASI Standard presently in existence that defines either the technical requirements for the criticality detection system, the reliability of the system, or the testing and calibration that should be performed.   The ANS-8 Subcommittee has prepared a Standard that is to be issued as a USASI Standard.

The paper mentioned above by Mr. Aspinall contains a significant amount of technical data upon which to base the requirements of a Criticality Detection and Alarm System.   He suggests that "neutron detection, with gamma insensitivity should be sought because neutron surge will normally be that characteristic of a fission chain most likely to differentiate it from other phenomena."   He discusses the detection threshold for both gamma and neutron detectors and the response time necessary to respond to the pulse.   He suggests that "detection should be of an increment of dose rate" rather than an increment of dose.   However, the subject of reliability received little attention.   He further suggested that the thoughtful choice of evacuation routes and the size of the evacuation area are important.

The draft copy of the ANS-USASI Standard, "Criticality Accident Alarm System" included the following suggested features for a system:

1. Detectors
    Gamma-ray rate meters

2. Alarm Set Point
    50 mR/hr

3. Coincidence
    Activation of at least two instruments required for alarm.

4. Detector Spacing
    Detectors located so that no point in the area to be covered is more than 450 ft from a detector.   Spacing is adjusted to compensate for any massive shielding.

5. Alarms

Distinctive sounds produced by electrome-
chanical or gas-driven devices having a
rapid response time (bells, Klaxons, air
horns, or public address systems). Remote
manual resets provided.

6. Reliability

System tests to be conducted weekly until
sufficient confidence has been developed to
permit the test schedule to be relaxed.

BNWL DESIGN CRITERIA

Spurious false criticality alarm signals have
plagued most plants using fissionable materials at
one time or another. These false signals have also
been experienced at Battelle with an average annual
frequency of eight occurrences. Since false alarms
were occurring from a number of causes, not all of
which were known, an investigating committee was
established to determine what measures could be
taken to reduce these false alarms, and, at the same
time, to alter the existing system to meet the license
requirements of 10 CFR 70.

With this background in mind, the radiological
instrument development group went to work on the
design of an improved criticality detector which would
provide the needed reliability. The following design
criteria were established by the steering committee
of radiation protection personnel and design engineers
for the proposed system:

1. Detectors—neutron sensitive and insensitive
to gamma radiation at levels up to 1000 R/hr;
alarm trip point between 10 and 1000 mrem/hr
above background; and shall not saturate when
subjected to an intense radiation field.

2. Relay and power control units—detectors wired for "2-out-of-n" operation (n≥3); all criticality alarm systems provided with emergency power; wiring shall be run in conduits used only for criticality detector leads; and a regulated and filtered power supply.

3. Audible alarms—a unique audible alarm used only to signal immediate evacuation from a criticality; a minimum of two alarm horns audible from any location where a criticality might occur;* and the minimum sound level of the alarm horns is 65 db in all normally occupied areas where a criticality might occur.

As noted, reliability of performance was uppermost in the overall design of this criticality detection system.   The high degree of dependability was based on the use of (1) a proven neutron detector, (2) an "internal" (fail-safe) audit circuit, (3) emergency power, and (4) a "2-out-of-n" detector-alarm matrix.

BNWL SYSTEM

The criticality detector was described by P. C. Friend at a previous Health Physics meeting. A few of the more important features of the system are included to provide an integrated view of the whole system. The detectors, which are adjustable so that the trip point for an alarm can be set at various neutron dose rates have been tested at dose rates between 18 and 700 mrem/hr. Any increase of a few mrem/hr across the trip point will cause an alarm. The trip time will vary from fractions of a second to a couple

---

*At BNW, any building in which greater than 1/3 of a minimum critical mass of fissionable material is permitted must have a criticality alarm system.

of seconds depending on the rate of change of dose
rate regardless of the trip point chosen. The system
will respond to a neutron burst as short as 50 μsec.

The detector-trip circuit package is mounted in
a metal case 11 x 11 x 8 inches. A system of colored
lights is mounted on each detector to indicate its
operating status; Normal, Audit Failure, or Criticality
Trip. Signals indicating abnormal conditions, i.e.,
criticality trip or audit failure, are transmitted to a
central comparator unit in each facility. Any abnormal
condition signal from the detector units will annunciate at the comparator, and remotely at a continuously manned central power-control panel. Criticality
trip signals from two or more detector units will,
in addition, set off the criticality alarms within the
building and annunciate remotely at the central emergency headquarters.

PERFORMANCE

The neutron detectors have been in service using
a 1-out-of-1 system for two years during which time
only six false alarms occurred principally as a result of line transients. (This major cause has been
overcome in the latest version which incorporates
line filters, isolation transformers, and wiring in
isolated conduits.) During the last eight months, the
coincidence circuitry has been employed without any
false alarms.

Detectors set to trip at 20 mrem/hr were tested
at the Oak Ridge Health Physics Research Reactor
and at the Sandia Pulsed Reactor Facility. At Oak
Ridge, the detectors, located on the far side of a hill

from the pulsed reactor, detected neutrons that
scattered over the hill and then passed through shielding of from one to three feet of concrete at distances
of greater than 400 feet. Gamma sensitive detectors,
located identically, did not detect the bursts. At
Sandia, where the flat desert terrain matches that of
the Richland location, units within a radius of 1150
feet of the shielded pulsed reactor detected the smal-
lest burst that the Sandia reactor has generated to
date, 1.27 x 10^{15} fissions. Larger bursts were
detected as far away as 1900 feet. During these tests
the reactor was shielded with 1 inch of polyethylene,
1 inch of boron, 7 inches of gypsum, and 54 inches of
concrete.

These measurements imply a dose rate of greater
than 100 mrem/hr at 500 feet from a burst (in a metal
system) of 10^{15} fissions with a shield between the
burst and detector of greater than the equivalent of
5 feet of concrete. From these test results, it appears
quite possible that all detector units in the main
Pacific Northwest Laboratory area (~0.25 square
mile) would trip if a criticality occurred anywhere
in the area.

To check sensitivity at trip points greater than
20 mrem/hr, theoretical calculations were made
using the following assumptions:

1. Minimum criticality accidents to be detected—
    10^{14} fissions (metal), 10^{15} fissions (moder-
    ated).

2. One neutron released per fission.

3. Source-to-detector distance (max.)—300 ft.

4. Shielding the equivalent 12 inches of normal concrete between source and detector.

Therefore, a criticality of 10^{14} fissions in a metallic system would result in a minimum neutron dose rate at the detector (300 ft) of 900 mrem/hr. For a moderated system, a criticality involving 10^{15} fissions would give a minimum neutron dose rate of 140 mrem/hr at the detector (300 ft).

Based on the above results and assumed conditions, the existing neutron sensitive criticality detectors will respond to a minimum criticality burst, be it moderated or not, when the alarm trip point is less than or equal to 100 mrem/hr and the detectors are within 300 feet of the burst. Therefore, instruments exhibiting these sensitivities can be expected to cover as much as a 300 ft radius in a fissionable material handling or storage area in the event of a minimum criticality.

Table I provides a comparison of the Battelle-Northwest Criticality Detection System to the proposed ANS-USASI Standard.

With the exception of the detector, the Battelle-Northwest system is comparable to one that would meet the proposed ANS-USASI Standard and should meet the "fail-safe" requirements stated in Mr. Aspinall's article. The requirement for a gamma detector appears to be unrealistic since neutrons may be a better indication of an accidental criticality than gamma rays. Perhaps this requirement is related to the availability of neutron detectors?

Certainly our solution (using neutron detectors) is not unique, but, can be or has been repeated a number of times througout the nuclear industry. It

Table I

	ANS-USASI*	BNW
Reliability	Weekly	Hourly
Detector	Gamma-Dose Rate	Neutron-Dose Rate
Minimum Response Time	1 msec	50 μsec
Alarm Set Point	50 mR/hr	100 mrem/hr
Coincidence	2-out-of-n	2-out-of-n
Maximum Detector Spacing	450 feet	300 feet

*From Appendix A of Standard which is provided as an example.

would appear that the technology has developed to the extent that the USASI Standard should be adopted and federal regulations should be written which will encourage the improvement of criticality detection systems to the point where they are truly the "last ditch defense designed to operate when all else has failed."

ACKNOWLEDGEMENT

The authors wish to acknowledge P. C. Friend, R. C. Weddle and L. V. Zuerner, the designers of the Battelle-Northwest Neutron Criticality Detection System.

BIBLIOGRAPHY

AEC Manual Chapter Appendix, "Safety of AEC-Owned Reactors".

Code of Federal Regulations, Title 10, Section 70.

P.C. Friend, "Burst Reactor Tests of a Neutron Sensitive Criticality Detector", BNWL-CC-1834, September 30, 1968.

USA Standard, "Immediate Evacuation Signal".

ANS 8.3 (Proposed Standard) "Criticality Accident Alarm System.

K. J. Aspinall, "Criticality Detection and Alarm Systems", Nuclear Engineering, March 1966.

PROGRESS ON SURFACE CONTAMINATION STANDARDS

F. E. Gallagher
California Institute of Technology
Pasadena, California
A. N. Tschaeche
General Electric Company
San Jose, California
C. A. Willis
McDonnell Douglas Corporation
Santa Monica, California
J. C. Evraets
University of California at Los Angeles
Los Angeles, California
J. C. Rogers
Los Angeles County Health Department
Los Angeles, California

ABSTRACT

A surface contamination standard is being developed, based on the following principles:

1. Non-zero permissible surface contamination limits should be based on health and safety criteria.

2. The standard must include limits for controlled and uncontrolled areas. These are not necessarily proportional to each other.

3. The standard must be constructed around the consideration that the limits chosen for uncontrolled areas may become a universal level of contamination.

4. Fallout, the major source of data for environmental contamination, indicates that the principle path to man is foodstuff contamination. Uncontrolled area limits should, therefore, be based upon data obtained from studies of radioactive fallout from weapons testing.

5. The limits should be selected so that surface contamination produces only a fraction (perhaps 10%) of the permissible dose.

6. Special cases, such as a plutonium dispersal following a weapons accident may require a different set of limits than those derived from fallout levels in uncontrolled areas.

7. Administrative controls need not be based on hazard, but may take into consideration such requirements as clean low level counting rooms, etc.

BACKGROUND

An ad hoc committee of the Southern California Chapter of the Health Physics Society was established several years ago to encourage the development of

radiation protection standards. During the second
organizational meeting of this committee, held on
December 12, 1967, several smaller ad hoc committees were formed to write specific standards. Our
group tentatively chose the topic of surface contamination
limits. A mail questionaire had been distributed to local
health physicists before the second meeting and general
surface contamination limits received the highest number of positive responses of the twenty nine suggested
topics. Subsequently, the national Health Physics
Society Standards Committee requested that we write
a standard for surface contamination limits in operational facilities.

At our first organizational meeting in the summer
of 1968, we decided to start with a position paper in
which we would state our basic position and ground rules
prior to actually writing the standard. We also decided
not to restrict our efforts to operational facilities, but
to include uncontrolled areas as well. The rest of this
paper is a tentative draft of our position paper, including
certain areas in which we need to make additional decisions before submitting our final draft to the Board
of Directors.

INTRODUCTION

Guidelines for both external and internal radiation
exposure have been developed by the International Commission on Radiological Protection. In the United States,
these have been supplemented by reports of the National
Committee on Radiological Protection and the Federal
Radiation Council. Under the U.S. Atomic Energy Act
of 1954 (68 Stat 919), as amended, the U.S. Atomic

Energy Commission has established two detailed sets of regulations: (1) The A. E. C. Manual for A. E. C. contractors, and (2) Title 10 of the Code of Federal Regulations for A. E. C. licensees. In addition, a number of states have entered into agreements with the A. E. C. to establish and enforce their own regulations, compatible of course with those of the A. E. C. , for certain amounts and types of radioactive material. Many states also regulate radiation producing machines independent of the A. E. C. agreements.

In order to demonstrate compliance with the regulations and the often conflicting interpretations of them, the reactor operator or radioisotope user must specify many details of operation. These are usually in the form of radiation safety manuals and operating procedures. These documents, almost without exception, define a set of surface contamination limits which apply to property under the control of the user. If a known quantitative relationship existed between surface contamination and internal radiation exposure, the task of setting these limits would be simple and straightforward. Since, this relationship is neither unique nor well known, establishing limits has been largely a subjective process. Organizations have adopted limits, based on a wide variety of criteria, with quite diversified results. Factors influencing a particular set of limits include:

(1) The philosophy of the facility management and their health physics personnel.

(2) The philosophy of the A. E. C. or state regulatory agency.

(3) The design of operational equipment and safe-
     guards.

(4) The actual degree of hazard present.

EXISTING AND RECOMMENDED LIMITS

One of the general categories of surface contamination limits is use today is the concept that "zero" or
"no detectable" contamination is the only acceptable
level for uncontrolled areas. Unfortunately, the minimum detectable activity depends on the sensitivity of
the survey meter or counting equipment used to measure the contamination. This quantity may vary widely
between different detectors, shielding arrangements,
and electronic discrimination. There are radioactive
materials present in our environment, both naturally
occurring nuclides such as ^{40}K, ^{226}Ra, and ^{222}Rn,
and artificially created isotopes such as ^{137}Cs, ^{90}Sr,
and other long-lived fission products. These can be
detected rather easily almost anywhere. Are we to
require cleanup of these contaminants or are we going
to specify that surface contamination may only be measured with certain less sensitive instruments? Instead
of basing limits on an arbitrary counting system, this
committee feels that these limits should be based on
the hazard represented by the particular isotope and
amount of radioactive material present.

Report No. 30 of the National Committee on
Radiation Protection[1] contains suggested levels of
"significant contamination" and factors which modify
these limits. The limits are based on meter response
and are as follows:

Measuring Instruments	Level for Nuclides in group	
	1 and 2	3 and 4
Geiger counter (β,γ)	100 cpm	100 cpm
Ionization Chamber	0.1 mrad/hr	0.1 mrad/hr
Alpha counter	1 dpm/cm^2	10 dpm/cm^2

The nuclides in each group are listed in the report. Group 1 includes the most radiotoxic materials such as ^{239}Pu and ^{90}Sr, while the other groups contain less radiotoxic material. Modifying factors for these limits which are listed include,

(1) The relative hazard of the radionuclide involved, including both external radiation and uptake in the body.

(2) The degree of fixation of the contaminant.

(3) The mobility of the article involved.

(4) The accessibility of the contamination in the normal use of the article.

(5) The possible interference with sensitive radiation measurements.

These levels of contamination and modifying factors are used primarily to establish a level at which contaminated items can receive an "unconditional release from control".

The recently published regulations of the U. S. Department of Transportation[2] contain a section on surface contamination limits for packages of radioactive material. These limits are for removable contamination as measured on the wiping material, and are:

(1) For all radionuclides except natural or depleted uranium and natural thorium,

   (a) 220 dpm/100 cm^2 for alpha contamination.

   (b) 2,200 dpm/100 cm^2 for beta-gamma contamination.

(2) For natural or depleted uranium and natural thorium,

   (a) 2,200 dpm/100 cm^2 for alpha contamination.

   (b) 22,000 dpm/100 cm^2 for beta-gamma contamination.

They do not have any limits for fixed contamination on the exterior of the package, however there are dose rate limits for each package, which would include fixed beta-gamma contamination, of 200 mrem/hour at the surface and 10 mrem/hour at three feet.

The Chicago Operations Office of the U.S. Atomic Energy Commission[3] has proposed a set of surface contamination limits for the release from control of decommissioned reactor sites. The limits for removable contamination are very similar to the recently adopted regulations of the Department of Transportation. They are:

(1) 1,000 dpm/100 cm^2 for the alpha emitters Nat U, ^{235}U, ^{238}U, Nat. Th, ^{232}Th, and associated decay products.

(2) 100 dpm/100 cm^2 for all other alpha emitters.

(3) 1,000 dpm/100 cm^2 for all beta-gamma emitters.

However, this A. E. C. Proposal also contains a series of limits for total contamination that is, fixed and removable combined. There are two independent sets of limits, one is basically ten times the removable contamination limits for alpha emitters and 0.4 mrad/hour at one centimeter for beta-gamma emitters. The other set permits higher maximum levels but slightly lower average levels (2.5 times and 0.5 times the first limits respectively). There are several footnotes with these limits describing the conditions, limitations, and definitions which interpret their use.

There have been attempts to calculate surface contamination limits based on the hazards of internal exposure, although much of the experimental data remains poorly defined and incomplete. One example of this approach is that used by Dunster[4,5] to derive the surface contamination limits normally used in the United Kingdom. These limits are related to airborne contamination by means of a resuspension factor obtained in part by theory and based partially on experimental data. The actual recommended limits are those for the more toxic emitters, with simplifying assumptions and rounding off. These limits apply to removable contamination and the health physicist within a facility is authorized to relax the limits for fixed contamination at his discretion. The limits that Dunster recommends are:

(1) For controlled areas

   (a) 22,000 dpm/100 cm^2 for the more toxic alpha emitters.

   (b) 220,000 dpm/100 cm^2 for certain less toxic alpha emitters such as uranium, thorium, and short-lived nuclides such as radon daughters.

(c) 220,000 dpm/100 cm^2 for beta emitters.

(2) For uncontrolled areas

    (a) 2,200 dpm/100 cm^2 for the more toxic alpha emitters.

    (b) 22,000 dpm/100 cm^2 for the same less toxic alpha emitters mentioned above.

    (c) 22,000 dpm/100 cm^2 for beta emitters.

These limits are quite liberal when compared to most surface contamination limits used in the United States.

In an independent attempt to mathematically derive a set of surface contamination limits based on the hazards of radiation exposure, Spangler and Willis[6, 7] calculated a permissible contamination level for each isotope, based on internal exposure, external gamma exposure, and external beta exposure. They then simplified the results to six different isotope groups with further relaxation permitted for six individual nuclides in controlled areas. Surface contamination limits for uncontrolled areas are proposed which are based on the fallout levels observed at that time. The limits they propose are:

(1) For controlled areas

    (a) 50 dpm/100 cm^2 for completely unknown mixtures of radionuclides

    (b) 100 dmm/100 cm^2 if none of the following radionuclides is present: ^{231}Pa, Nat Th, ^{239}Pu, 240Pu, ^{242}Pu, and ^{249}Cf.

    (c) 200 dpm/100 cm^2 if none of the following radionuclides is present: ^{227}Ac, ^{230}Th,

^{232}Th, ^{238}Pu, ^{231}Pa, Nat Th, ^{239}Pu, ^{240}Pu, ^{242}Pu, and ^{249}Cf.

(d) 1,000 dpm/100 cm^2 if none of the following radionuclides is present: ^{237}Np, ^{252}Cf, ^{250}Cf, ^{246}Cm, ^{245}Cm, ^{243}Cm, ^{241}Am, ^{228}Th, ^{244}Cm, ^{232}U, ^{227}Ac, ^{230}Th, ^{232}Th, ^{238}Pu, ^{231}Pa, Nat Th, ^{239}Pu, ^{240}Pu, ^{242}Pu, and ^{249}Cf.

(e) 10,000 dpm/100 cm^2 if no alpha emitting radionuclides are present.

(f) 40,000 dpm/100 cm^2 if no alpha emitting radionuclides are present and ^{90}Sr and ^{129}I are not present.

(g) 50,000 dpm/100 cm^2 for ^{3}H and ^{22}Na.

(h) 70,000 dpm/100 cm^2 for ^{65}Zn.

(i) 10^7 dpm/100 cm^2 for ^{14}C and ^{35}S.

(2) For uncontrolled areas, the levels vary between 1,000 dpm/100 cm^2 and 10,000 dpm/100 cm^2, depending on the toxicity of the particular nuclides involved, determined from a curve constructed by the authors.

PROPOSALS FOR A SURFACE
CONTAMINATION STANDARD

Our ad hoc committee studying surface contamination standards believes that enough evidence is available, relating surface contamination with health hazard, to allow the establishment of a standard, perhaps through the U.S.A. Standards Institute. While many organizations, such as Oak Ridge National Laboratory, Los Alamos Scientific Laboratory, and many others, have operational limits which have been in effect for many years, a standard will be particularly valuable to the smaller facilities which do not have a long history of health physics activities. There are many schools and industries in the United States which use relatively small amounts of activity, often of the less radiotoxic nuclides, that could use a standard such as this one in setting up a meaningful radiation protection program. If the Society does not write this standard on a national scale, then the regulatory agencies will do it on a state by state basis; indeed, this may have already started.

The completed standard should consist of two sets of limits for general use. The first category includes controlled areas within operational facilities. Within this type of area access is generally limited to radiation workers, surveys of dose rates and surface contamination are conducted on a routine basis, eating and smoking are prohibited, and the use of radiation sources is under the supervision of a radiation protection officer and/or committee. These limits should be based on two concepts: (1) Beta and gamma dose rates; and (2) The Maximum Permissible Concentration in air, with a suitable resuspension factor to account for potential internal deposition of radioactive material. These limits would have to be flexible enough so that the facility health physicist could relax them when necessary, if additional safeguards such as coveralls and shoe covers were required.

The other set of limits should be for uncontrolled areas, either within operational facilities or in public

areas outside of operational facilities. For these
values, the only data that we have is studies of the
nature and effects of radioactive fallout from weapons
tests. Fallout is the only good source of information
that exists concerning the effects of low levels of environmental contamination on humans beings and
animals. The Federal Radiation Council[8] has stated
that,

(1) Present levels are acceptable.

(2) At the current fallout levels, foodstuff contami-
     nation is the dominant factor in human exposure.

(3) Present levels of ^{90}Sr contamination of ap-
     proximately 1,000 dpm/100 cm^2 are observed.

In addition, gross fission product activity levels are
much higher than the ^{90}Sr levels.[9] The standard
should be based on these statements.

The contamination limits should be selected so that
surface contamination produces only a fraction of the
maximum permissible dose: 10% has been chosen as a
convenient fraction for design purposes. Since the radiotoxicity of the various radionuclides is not equal, a wide
range of limit values may be appropriate. We have not,
however, decided whether or not to have broad groups
of radioactive materials with a limit for each group,
or to have a separate limit for each individual radionuclide. Several classifications of the radiotoxicity
already exist—two examples are: (1) the four toxicity
classes of the International Atomic Energy Agency; and
(2) the seven transport classes of the recently adopted
Department of Transportation regulations. Since surface contamination limits are often used in the field, the
definition of only a few categories may lead to easier

enforcement. A decision also must be made concerning external dose rates—should we have a set number of millirem per hour at a specified distance from a contaminated surface coupled with a value for removable contamination based on internal exposure hazards, or should we include both factors into a total contamination limit? We must decide these fundamental questions before we write the actual standard.

One serious problem with a surface contamination standard is the tendency of regulatory agencies to adopt standards and recommendations as part of their regulations. This has happened many times in the past history of health physics. Credible accidents could produce conditions wherein the application of a surface contaimination standard might be impractical. After a reactor excursion or plutonium dispersal following the crash of a bomber armed with nuclear weapons, the degree of decontamination becoms a matter which requires the judgement of many health physics and governmental personnel. We do not think that the levels left in Palomares, Spain would be suitable for Central Park in New York City. We may attempt to write the standard with suggestions for these unpleasant accidents. We will decide this before completing the position paper. There will certainly be zones where the suggested limits may be too high, such as low background counting facilities and whole body counters. Administrative controls, based on scientific requirements rather than personnel hazards, can easily handle these special cases. The standard will not consider these administrative controls, but will leave them entirely to the judgement of the appropriate project management.

CONCLUSION

A standard for surface contamination limits is
needed in the United States and an ad hoc committee has
been formed to write it. The first step is the preparation of a draft for a position paper describing what we
propose to include in the standard. The position paper
consists of a review of existing and proposed limits
and a description of what the committee feels is pertinent to include in the standards. Several questions
are asked in this paper, in areas where the committee would like to obtain feedback from the Society.
The limits chosen must be based on safety, utility of
enforcement, and sound health physics principles.
Please feel free to let us know any comments and suggestions that you feel would be of value in this project.

REFERENCES

1. "Safe Handling of Radioactive Materials," Recommendations of the National Committee on Radiation Protection, Report No. 30, NBS Handbook
   92, U.S. Department of Commerce, March 1964.

2. Hazardous Materials Regulations Board, U.S.
   Department of Transportation, "Radioactive
   Materials and Other Miscellaneous Amendments,"
   Federal Register, 33: 194, October 4, 1968.

3. J. L. Smith, "Proposed Contamination Levels for
   Release of Property at PNPF," A.E.C. Memorandum to K. A. Dunbar, Manager, Chicago Operations Office, U.S.A.E.C., April 12, 1968.

4. H. J. Dunster, "Surface Contamination Measurements as an Index of Control of Radioactive Materials," Health Physics, 8, August 1962.

5. H. J. Dunster, "Control Criteria for Radioactive Surface Contamination," Surface Contamination; Proceedings of an International Symposium, Gatlinburg, Tenn., June 1964," Pergamon Press, 1967.

6. G. W. Spangler and C. A. Willis, "Permissible Contamination Limits, "Surface Contamination; Proceedings of an International Symposium, Gatlinburg, Tenn., June 1964," Pergamon Press, 1967.

7. G. W. Spangler and C. A. Willis, "Permissible Contamination Limits: Values for Uncontrolled Areas and Some Special Cases," Presented at the Health Physics Society Annual Meeting, Los Angeles, Calif., June 1965.

8. Federal Radiation Council, "Estimates and Evaluation of Fallout in the United States from nuclear Weapons Testing Through 1962," FRC-4, May 1962.

9. L. Van Middlesworth, "Easily Measure Radioactive Fallout," Health Physics, 10, July 1964.

INTERNAL DOSIMETRY
PROBLEMS, DEFINITIONS & STANDARDS

A. N. Tschaeche
General Electric Company
San Jose, California

INTRODUCTION

The primary purpose of an internal dosimetry program is to protect individuals from excessive exposure to internal radiation. Acceptable protection is obtained when internal dose equivalents are kept below the levels recommended by the International Commission on Radiological Protection (ICRP). In addition, regulatory agencies may impose limits, and remaining below those limits is generally accepted as providing the required protection.

However, the path from internal dose to some measurement which can be related to dose is torturous and ill defined. Experimental data are lacking in many areas along this path. Relations between various parts of the path are extremely complex. It is time consuming and difficult to relate an internal dosimetric measurement to internal dose even when the path is known and the data extant.

1783

Therefore, even if the guides and regulations on internal dose were unambigous and simple, the problem of verifying that those guides or regulations were followed is severe. The health physicist is charged with this verification. He must present programs for internal dosimetry to his management to provide this verification. These programs are costly.

It is the purpose of this paper to demonstrate some of the problems the manager of an internal dosimetry program will face, to clarify the terms used in internal dosimetry and to show some of the guides and standards which are needed for implementation of optimum internal dosimetry programs.

THE PROBLEMS

Three major problems face a manager who must implement an internal dosimetry program.

1. There is great discrepancy between regulatory agencies in the limits and requirements for internal dosimetry.

2. There are no guides or standards upon which to base a logically sound internal dosimetry program without a large amount of expert help.

3. Internal dosimetry is expensive. Without guides, standards or regulations there is a strong tendency for cost rather than radiation protection to be the predominant consideration in developing an internal dosimetry program.

REGULATIONS ON INTERNAL DOSIMETRY

The first duty of the radiation protection manager is to protect people. His next duty is to see that laws are obeyed. Unfortunately, many managers will think too much about laws and not enough about people. Let us examine the laws which exist concerning internal dosimetry. Consider only the <u>letter</u> of the law, not the intent.

First, what internal dose limits exist in the regulations?

Table 1 shows a comparison of internal dose limits for three regulations and one guide (as of 2/69). The ICRP recommendations are included only for comparison since they are not law in this country. However other countries include in their laws provisions that recommendations of the ICRP should automatically apply.[1] External radiation dose equivalent limits are included for interest. Several things are significant about these numbers.

1.   There are no internal dose limits in California at all. This fact comes from the words of the law. All the dose limits are given under a paragraph titled "Occupational Dose Limits from <u>External</u> Exposure".

2.   10 CFR 20 has limits only for whole body, gonads, head and trunk, and active blood forming organs. There is also a lens of the eye limit which is much too restrictive compared with ICRP guides.

3.   Only the AEC Manual has limits which even begin to compare with the ICRP guides.

In addition to the limits in Table I, Table II shows a comparison of what I would interpret as the <u>meaning</u>

TABLE I

Some Current (1969) Guides & Regulations for Internal Dose Equivalent (Dose) Limits
Under Normal Circumstances

Organ	Lifetime Dose (rem)	Ave. Annual Dose (rem)	Max. Quarterly Dose (rem)
Whole Body	5(N-18), I*, CFR	5, I, AEC, CFR	3, I, AEC, CFR
Red Bone Marrow	5(N-18), I	5, I	3, I
Active Blood Forming Organs	-	5, AEC	3, AEC
	-	5, CFR	1 1/4, CFR
Head & Trunk	-	5, CFR	1 1/4, CFR
Gonads	5(N-18), I	5, I, AEC	3, I, AEC
	-	5, CFR	1 1/4, CFR
Lens of Eye	-	15, I	8, I
	-	15, AEC	5, AEC
	-	5, CFR	1 1/4, CFR
Thyroid	-	30, I	15, I
	-	30, AEC	10, AEC
Bone	-	30, I	15, I
	-	Body Burden of 0.1µg of Ra-226 or equivalent, AEC	
All Other Organs	-	15, I	8, I
	-	15, AEC	5, AEC
External Radiation			
Skin	-	30, I	15, I
	-	30, AEC	10, AEC
	-		7 1/4, CFR, C**
Extremities	-	75, I	38, I
	-	75, AEC	30, AEC
	-		18 3/4, CF

*   I - International Commission on Radiological Protection[2]
    AEC - Atomic Energy Commission Manual For Prime Contractors[3]
     CFR - 10 CFR 20 for AEC Licensees[4]
**   C - California Radiation Regulations[5]

TABLE II

Comparison of Current (1969) Guides & Regulations
for Internal Dose Equivalent
(Dose) Measurements

Organization		Requirement for Internal Dose Measurement*
ICRP	1.	All organs#[6] (if might exceed 0.3 x annual limit)[7]
	2.	Can control on air & water concentrations also[8]
AEC	1.	All organs#[9]
	2.	Can control on air & water concentrations also[10]
	3.	Must report annually all people who have annual average exposure[11] of >1/2 MPBB-year (or MPOB-year)
10 CFR 20	1.	Whole body, head & trunk, active blood forming[12] organs, lens of eye, gonads
	2.	Must control air & water concentrations[13]
	3.	Availability of bioassay services to an individual may be directed by license condition[14]
CAC-17	1.	None
	2.	Must control air & water concentrations[15]
	3.	User shall make provision for regular bioassay program where indicated[16] by and appropriate to nature of potential exposure (sometimes license conditions imposed for bioassay).

*It is assumed that, if a limit is given, measurement to assure that limit is not exceeded is required.

All organs means all organs for which a limit is given by the organization as listed.

NOTE: See Appendix A for quotations on which this table was based.

of the letter of the laws on measurement requirements
for internal dosimetry.   Appendix A contains the actual
words of each law quoted.   ICRP recommendations are
again included for comparison.   In using Table I to
arrive at the conclusion in Table II, I made on in-
ference: if a limit is given in Table I measurement
must be made.

From Table II it may be seen that:

1.   The ICRP and AEC Manual require measurement of all internal doses.   The ICRP suggests measurements if dose might be above three-tenths of any
limit.[7] The AEC annual reporting requirement im-
poses some lower limit on measurements, but the
limit depends on the conditions of exposure.

2.   10 CFR 20 requires internal dose measurements for "whole body" type exposures.   In addition,
license conditions may require a bioassay program.

3.   California has no internal dose measurement
requirements.   Licenses are required to make provision for appropriate bioassay programs.   In addition some licenses are issued with specific bioassay
requirements.

4.   Of course the primary bastion of defense
against internal exposure is to keep radioactive material from being inhaled, ingested or otherwise entering
the body.   Therefore the ICRP and the AEC say that
concentrations of radioactive material in air and
water can and should be controlled.   For all licensees this control is mandatory.

After examining Tables I and II, it is easy to see
that the regulations do not offer much guidance for
internal dose limits and none at all for measurement

programs.   Even the ICRP has no help for the latter
problem.

DEFINITIONS

Before we continue, let us consider some of the
terms used in internal dosimetry and their definitions.
To aid in visualizing the relations between terms, Fig.
I shows a diagram of the components which make up
internal dosimetry and their relationship to each other.
The list of definitions is given in Appendix B.

The whole, over-all task of determining dose
equivalent may be called Internal Dosimetry.   This
includes measurements of radioactive material as well
as calculation of dose taking into account disintegra-
tion energy, half-life and quality factors, etc.

The ICRP used a new term in ICRP-9, Dose Commitment.[17] The idea is that, once the radioactive
material is inside a person, he is committed to it
based on the effective half-life.   And he will be committed to receive a dose equivalent until it is all gone.

There are two kinds of limit defined for internal
dose: the old standby as shown in Table I, and the relatively new limit recommended by the ICRP (1965) for
acute exposures, the Permitted Annual Maximum Dose
Commitment, for which I have coined the term PAMDO.
PAMDO is the dose equivalent which would result from
body intake by a person exposed for one year at the
maximum permissible concentration.

For example:

The 40-hr MPC for "soluble" Sr-90 is 40 x 1 x
10^{-9} μCi/cc (according to 10 CFR 20) or 4 x 10^{-8}

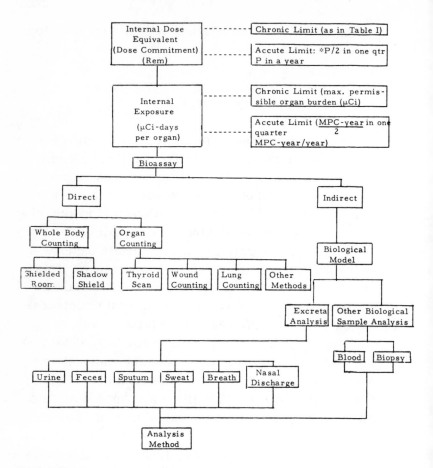

*PAMDO (See Appendix B for definition)

Fig. I. Components of Internal Dosimetry.

μCi-hrs/cc. 50 weeks at this concentration would be an MPC-year of 2 x 10^{-6} μCi-hrs/cc-year. Exposure to one MPC-year would result in a dose equivalent (integrated over 50 years because Sr-90 has a long effective half life) to the bone (the critical organ) of 30 rem. PAMDO would be 30 rem.

The ICRP recommends a quarterly limit of PAMDO/2 for single exposures. Dr. K. Z. Morgan presented an excellent summary of the new ICRP recommendations (which include PAMDO) at the 1965 Health Physics Society meeting in Los Angeles.[18]

Internal Exposure is reserved for the amount of radioactive material actually in the organ as a function of time. Exposure to radiation from radioactive material inside the body is the concern of internal dosimetry. Therefore, internal exposure to radioactive material for a given time results in an internal dose for that time.

The process of measuring something to arrive at internal exposure is called bioassay. Bioassay may be either direct, as whole body counting, or indirect, as analysing urine and using some model to relate excretion rate to amount of radioactive material in the organ at the time the sample was taken.

One may think of one bioanalysis as a snapshot of the situation at one instant in time. Then internal exposure is a movie of the situation over a period of time. It takes many bioassays for use in measuring internal exposure.

The other terms defined in Appendix B are self-explanatory and are needed for a reasonably complete list.

Let us now return to the manager, who must establish an internal dosimetry program, and consider how he might develop a basis or bases for his program.

INFORMATION NECESSARY FOR DEVELOPMENT
of Bases for Internal Dosimetry Program

In addition to the nomenclature, the manager must have knowledge of the following items:

1. The use(s) to which the internal dosimetric data are put.

2. The accuracy required for the uses and the factors which affect the accuracy.

3. The "state of the art" of measurements and data interpretation.

USES FOR INTERNAL DOSIMETRIC DATA

Internal dosimetry is used in a manner similar to external dosimetry.

1. To Check Routinely the Capability of Engineered Safeguards.

One wishes to assure that personnel are not exposed internally beyond the limits set during facility design. This use is similar to providing film badges to check external exposure after the fact (and for negative information for legal purposes).

2. Exposure Control

There may be times when one must control exposure by bioassay. AEC Contractors operating under Manual Chapter 0524 may do this occasionally. It is a very difficult thing to do and is not recommended; but when the necessity occurs, control usually is needed immediately. There is not time to do detailed analyses. Relatively detailed guides would be very helpful. This use is similar to employing film badges or pocket dosimeters to control external exposure.

3. Measurement

After a known intake of radioactive material (as in an accident) one needs to measure internal dose. This measurement is the most difficult of all. It corresponds to the kind of external dosimetry which is done after a criticality accident. People have been exposed, but their personnel monitors (film badges, etc.) don't tell the story. So detailed phantom measurements are made to determine the dose as accurately as possible. Naturally, the higher the dose, up to a point, the more carefully one need to measure. Beyond 10,000 rem it is rather academic. But at 500 rem or 20 organ burdens, it certainly is not.

In many cases routine checks result in the discovery of an internal exposure which requires measurement. Internal exposure control may also require dose measurement. Therefore the first two programs should be designed so that, at some indicated level of exposure, a measurement program is instituted.

4. Research

Accuracy The problem of accuracy is probably the most
difficult to define and resolve of all the problems in internal dosimetry.   Table III illustrates some of the
things which affect accuracy of various measurements
in the chain which leads to internal dose. In setting
up a program for one of the four reasons above, each
of these things needs to be considered. The list is not
exhaustive. It is intended only to illustrate the complexity of the problem. Only one factor in each suc-
ceeding step in the measurement of internal dose has
been amplified. The table would be rather large if
everything were shown.

It is clear that there are many, many factors
affecting the accuracy of the final dose number. It
would be helpful if recommended accuracies were already available. They are not. However data and
knowledgeable individuals exist so that accuracy
guides for annual internal doses could be established.

Accuracy for External Dose. Annual external exposure accuracy requirements have been suggested by at
least three people. Arthur R. Keene of BNW suggested[19] annual doses be accurate to $\pm 69\%$ at 2σ;
Franke & Hunzinger in Belgium suggest[20] $\pm 40\%$
based on genetic damage and $\pm 75\%$ based on life span
shortening; and Wheatley of England suggests[21] $\pm 50\%$
for estimating annual doses from dose rates, time
studies and other environmental monitoring methods
(not personnel monitoring). It is remarkable how
well these numbers agree.

Accuracy for Internal Dose. One might be arbitary
and say, "Very well, the accuracy required for annual

internal dose is ± 50% at 2 σ. " With that number, one has at least a starting point for everything else. One could assign or measure accuracies of all the other things that go into dose determination and, by judicious juggling get everything to balance properly.

An example may illustrate the kinds of problems accuracy requirements involve.

An inhalation incident occurred a few years ago with which the author was involved. The radioactive material was non-translocatable so the lung was the critical organ. There were strong indications that the MPC's of 10CFR20 were too high because the material had an effective half life in the lung of 300 days or more. Therefore, if exposure had been limited to 40 MPC hours per week, the maximum permissible lung burden would have been exceeded. So the urine excretion rate was used to control exposure. However, it was estimated that some of the people had about one lung burden eventually. The question was— how accurately did the internal exposure have to be measured? That translated into:

1) How often do you need to sample?

2) How well do you need to know the actual daily urine output of each person?

3) Do you have to take 24-hour samples or do creatnine analysis to determine daily output?

4) What other measurements are necessary (e.g. whole body counting and fecal analysis)?

The amount of money involved in increased sampling and analysis could have been about $10,000. It is not certain exactly what increase in accuracy that

TABLE III

Some Factors Affecting Accuracy of an Internal Dosimetry Program

Things to be Determined	Things Measured or Estimated	Factors Affecting Measurement or Estimation Accuracy
A. Internal Dose Equivalent (rem)	1. Internal Exposure (μCi-days)	1. Measurement frequency 2. See B. below
	2. Quality factor(s) 3. Disintegration energy (mev) 4. Decay scheme (particles per disintegration) 5. Tissue distribution of radioactive material 6. Organ mass	Many
B. Internal Exposure (μCi-days)	1. Effective half life	1. Excretion rate 2. Translocation rate 3. Radionuclide half life
	2. Nuclide fractionation (Am-241--Pu-241)	1. Biological & chemical factors
	3. Amount of radioactive material in the organ	See C. below

C. Amount of Radioactive
Material in the Organ

I. Measured directly

1. Radiation coming out of organ

    1. Counter calibration
    2. Patient position
    3. Tissue absorption
    4. Background
    5. Relation between radiation measured & radiation of interest (e.g. U-235/U-234, Am-241/Pu-239
    6. Distribution of radioactive matl. in other parts of body.

II. Measured indirectly

1. Amount of radioactive material in excreta

    1. Variations in daily excretion rate
    2. Relation of sample taken to daily total excreted
    3. Method of sample analysis
    4. Variations in amount of excreta per day

2. Biological model used to relate amount excreted to amount in organ

    1. Many

expenditure would have bought. It might have made a difference of a factor between 2 and 5 in determining internal exposure. Whether that factor was important was not established.

However, the determinations were not made and sampling frequency was actually reduced although some other measurements were made. Management could not see spending a large amount of money if it could not be convinced logically that the expenditure was necessary. It was not enough to say that it would be nice to have the numbers. Management said that the company was not in the research business. And they were right! But no one could give them a logical and convincing argument that accuracy greater than that they already had was necessary without a long and expensive examination of the "state of the art" of internal dosimetry. There was not even a guide. Perhaps help might have been found in the literature, but a literature search would have cost money, too. The management of this company would have been greatly aided if it had been able to refer to an easily-applied guide on which to base its internal dosimetric sampling program.

BASES FOR INTERNAL
DOSIMETRY PROGRAMS

The uses for internal dosimetry, the accuracy required and some factors affecting the accuracy have been briefly discussed. The state of the art of internal dosimetric measurement techniques and data interpretation will be passed over without comment, other than to say that they have improved in the past 20 years.

The question of bases for internal dosimetry programs may now be considered.

The first and most general use of internal dosimetry is in routine checking to see that engineered safeguards are really working. This kind of program usually uses urinalysis although fecal analysis and whole body counting are very necessary in some situations. Several bases for sampling frequency have been offered in the literature. The British offered one for plutonium.[21] West and Reavis of Oak Ridge[22] offered one of general applicability based on a probablistic approach and recent past bioassay data. Sanders and Knight of Savannah[23] developed a similar system which does not require knowledge of recent past history. There may be still others. No comment will be made on the worth of these systems. They are offered for information. These systems only indicate the minimum frequency of sampling. They do not say what to do if a non-zero result is obtained and subsequent results remain elevated. A guide would be helpful to act as part of the basis for a measurement program once an internal exposure has occurred, but the author knows of no published bases for such situations.

The cases of control and measurement likewise have a lack of published guides. There are data in many documents on individual cases. But there is no single place where one can find a basis for an internal dosimetry program for these uses. Fortunately, the control case doesn't occur very often and then usually only with AEC prime contractors who have some capability in this field. But the measurement case can and does grow out of the routine checking case quite frequently and is very important. Since internal dosimetric measurements increase in cost very rapidly with increase in accuracy requirements, this is the area where guidance would be very useful.

There is one guide which has been recently published by the ICRP, ICRP Publication 10,[25] which gives some help in relating urinary excretion rates to organ burdens. But it does not give much help in selecting sampling programs.

STANDARDS AND GUIDES

Table IV shows some areas where useful standards or guides whould be developed. The items listed under A, B, F and G could be standards. The others must be guides until more information is available.

One particular subject needs to be amplified—the standards and guides which apply to analysis of bioassay samples. Many radionuclide users rely on outside vendors to analyze samples. The problems of finding a vendor who performs analyses quickly and accurately are legion. These problems are of the same kind as those associated with film badge suppliers.

When one looks for a supplier, what bases are available on which to judge him? Is enough known about all the analyses methods for a particular nuclide to pick the best one? Are administrative procedures similar enough between suppliers to permit comparison? Does the user have the ability to spike samples so that the vendor's accuracy may be checked? How good does the vendor's accuracy have to be? How low do his detection limits have to be? It would save time and money, and hopefully produce more

TABLE IV

Standards or Guides Useful in Internal Dosimetry

A. Nomenclature & Definitions

B. Analysis Methods for Bioassay Samples
    1. Sr-90
    2. U-natural up to 5% enriched
    3. U-enriched >5%
    4. Plutonium
    5. Tritium
    6. Gross alpha
    7. Gross beta
    8. Mixed fission products
    9. Others (many)

C. Sampling Frequency for Various Internal Dosimetric Uses
    1. Routine sampling for engineered safeguards checking purposes.
    2. (a) To detect internal exposures
        (b) To estimate internal dose if exposure occurred.
    3. To control internal exposure
    4. To measure internal dose equivalent.

D. Kind of Sample Needed for Various Internal Dosimetric Programs
    1. Some conditions which influence sample kind
        (a) Nuclide
        (b) Nuclide type
             (1) Translocatable
             (2) Non-translocatable
        (c) Accuracy desired
        (d) Dosimetric use

E. Excreta Limits for Chronic & Accute Exposures for Various Nuclides
    nd Nuclide Types

F. ranslocatability of Various Chemical Compounds of Nuclides

G. Administrative Procedures in Indirect Bioassay Programs
    1. Sample identification methods
    2. Sample collection methods and hardware
    3. Sample handling techniques
        (a) Pre-treatment before analysis
        (b) Sample protection during shipment
    4. Records needed
    5. Education of operators, management, technicians (in bioassay program)
    6. Bioassay sample laboratory construction and administration.

H. Accuracy Needed for Various Dosimetric Uses
    1. Routine monitoring
        (a) for internal exposure detection
        (b) for internal dose estimation if exposure occurred
    2. Internal exposure control
    3. Measurement of internal dose equivalent.

accurate answers if there were standards to help
answer these questions.

SUMMARY

There remains two final points to consider. How
did this state of affairs come to exist? And is there
really a problem?

The state of affairs exists because the AEC, FRC,
NCRP and ICRP adopted the philosophy that internal
exposure is best controlled by limiting the exposure
to concentrations of radioactive material in air and
water. Because of the extremely complicated nature
of internal dosimetry, and the lack of knowledge in this
area, the philosophy was a good one. And the situation
has not been nor is serious at present. But three
things indicate a movement toward the direction of
potentially serious problems.

1. There are an increasing number of people
handling loose radioactive material.

2. There is increasing pressure to change concentration limits for radioactive material in air and
water from those averaged weekly to those averaged
quarterly or even yearly.

3. There is evidence to show that the AEC should
provide performance standards for safety rather than
detailed design standards.[26]

Any one of these reasons is sufficient to start a
program to improve internal dosimetry. When all
three occur at once, the program must be an accelerated one.

Therefore efforts must be made to develop guides and standards for internal dosimetry programs. These guides and standards are needed immediately to aid those who must have existing programs, and only slightly less immediately to help the larger number who will need such programs in the future. The health physics family and the nuclear industry should develop these standards and guides rather than wait for regulatory agencies to do it. After all, it is the nuclear industry itself which is primarily responsible for radiation safety.

REFERENCES

1. "Protection Against Ionizing Radiations", a survey of existing regulations, World Health Organization, Geneva, 1964, p. 10.

2. "Recommendations of the International Commission on Radiological Protection", ICRP Publication 9, p. 10, para. 56 (1965).

3. U.S. Atomic Energy Commission Manual Chapter 0524, "Standards for Radiation Protection", Appendix A, p. 3 (1963).

4. Title 10 Code of Federal Regulations, "Atomic Energy", Part 20, "Standards for Protection Against Radiation", Section 20.101, "Exposure of Individuals to Radiation in Restricted Areas", (1966).

5. California Administrative Code, Title 17, "Public Health", Chapter 5, Subchapter 4, "Radiation", Group 3, "Standards for Protection Against

Radiation", Article 3, "Dose Limits, Permissible Levels and Concentrations", Section 30265, "Occupational Dose Limits from External Exposure" (1968).

6. ICRP Publication 9, p. 10, para. 56 (1965).

7. ICRP Publication 9, p. 19, paragraphs 111, 112 (1965).

8. "Recommendations of the International Commission on Radiological Protection", Report of Subcommittee II on Permissible Dose for Internal Radiation, ICRP Publication 2, p. 4, para 2(c), (1959).

9. AEC Manual Chapter 0524, Appendix A, p. 3 para. I.B.2.

10. ibid, Appendix A, p. 3, para. I.B.1.

11. AEC Manual Chapter 0502.

12. Title 10 Code of Federal Regulations, "Atomic Energy", Part 20, "Standards for Protection Against Radiation", Section 20.101, "Exposure of Individuals to Radiation in Restricted Areas", (1966).

13. ibid, Section 20.103, "Exposure to Individuals to Concentrations of Radioactive Material in Restricted Areas", (1966).

14. ibid, Section 20.108, "Orders Requiring Furnishing of Bioassay Services", (1966).

15. California Administrative Code, Title 17, "Public Health", Chapter 5, Subchapter 4, "Radiation", Group 3, "Standards for Protection Against

Radiation", Article 3, "Dose Limits, Permissible Levels and Concentrations", Section 30266, "Exposure of Individuals to Concentrations of Radioactive Material in Controlled Areas", (1968).

16. ibid, Section 30277, "Bioassays and Medical Surveillance", (1968).

17. ICRP Publication 9, p. 10, para. 54.

18. K. Z. Morgan, "Present Status of Recommendations of the International Commission on Radiological Protection, National Council on Radiation Protection, and Federal Radiation Council", presented at the Annual Meeting of the Health Physics Society held in Los Angeles, California, June 14, 1964.

19. A. R. Keene, "Purposes, Required Accuracy and Interpretation of Personnel Monitoring", Symposium on Radiation Dose Measurements, Their Purpose, Interpretation and Required Accuracy in Radiological Protection, E. N. E. A. & A. E. P. E. N., p. 49, (1967).

20. Th. Franke & W. Hunsinger, "The Accuracy of Dosimetry Consistent with Variances in Biological Damage", Symposium on Radiation Dose Measurements, Their Purpose, Interpretation and Required Accuracy in Radiological Protection, E. N. E. A. and A. E. P. E. N., p. 261, (1967).

21. B. M. Wheatly, "Confidence Limits on Measurements in the Working Environment", Symposium on Radiation Dose Measurements, Their Purpose, Interpretation and Required Accuracy in Radiological Protection, E. N. E. A. & A. E. P. E. N., p. 415, (1967).

22. S. A. Beach, et al, "Basis for Routine Urine Sampling of Workers Exposed to Pu-239", Health Physics, 12, p. 1671 (1966) AHSB (RP)-R-68.

23. C. M. West & J. P. Reavis, "Use of Statistics in an Applied Health Physics Program", Health Physics, 10, #5, p. 345, (May 1964).

24. F. D. Knight & S. M. Saunders, Jr., "A Probabilistic Method of Appraising Bioassay Sampling Programs", Health Physics, 14 #5, p. 523 (May 1968).

25. ICRP Publication 10, "Evaluation of Radiation Doses to Body Tissues from Internal Contamination due to Occupational Exposure" (1968).

26. "Report to the Atomic Energy Commission by the Radioisotopes Licensing Review Panel", G. F. Trowbridge, Chairman, Sept. 5, 1967.

APPENDIX A

Regulations on Internal Dosimetry

A. AEC Manual Chapter 0524

Standards for Radiation Protection

I. Radiation Protection Standards for Individuals in Controlled Areas*

    A.

    B. Radiation from emitters internal to the body.

        1. Except as provided in 2 below, the radiation protection standards for airborne radioactivity specified in annex I, table I, shall be followed. The concentration standards are based upon continuous exposure to the concentrations specified for forty hours per week (a "week" being seven consecutive days). For the purpose of applying these standards, radioactivity concentrations may be averaged over periods up to 13 consecutive weeks provided work areas are appropriately monitored and exposure histories are maintained for each individual working in such areas.

        2. If it is not feasible to govern exposures to internal emitters by applying airborne

---

*An individual under age 18 shall not be employed in or allowed to enter controlled areas in such manner that he will receive doses of radiation in amounts exceeding the standards applicable to individuals in uncontrolled areas. Exposures to individuals under age 18 may be averaged over peiods not to exceed one calendar quarter.

radioactivity concentration standards, the
following radiation protection standards
shall apply:

Type of Exposure	Dose	
	rem/year	rem/quarter
Whole body, active bloodforming organs, gonads.	5	3
Thyroid	30	10
Bone	Body burden of 0.1 microgram of radium-226 or its biological equiv- alent*	
Other organs	15	5

B.   California Administrative Code, Title 17

Article 3. Dose Limits, Permissible Levels and
Concentrations.

30265. Occupational Dose Limits from External
Exposure. (a) Except as provided in Section
30265 (b), no user shall posses sources of radiation in such a manner as to cause (1) any individual 18 years of age or over to receive an occupational dose in excess of the limits specified in
the following table, or (2) any individual under 18
years of age to receive an occupational dose in

---

*Exposure must be governed such that the indi-
vidual's body burden does not exceed this value(a) when
averaged over any period of 12 consecutive months and
(b) after 50 years of occupational exposure.

excess of 10% of the limits specified in the following table:

	Rems per calendar quarter
Whole body	1.25
Hands and forearms; feet and ankles	18.75
Skin of the whole body	7.5

(b) A user may permit an individual 18 years of age or over to receive an occupational dose to the whole body greater than that permitted under Section 30265(a), provided that:

(1) during any calendar quarter the occupational dose to the whole body shall not exceed 3 rems;

30266.   Exposure of Individuals to Concentrations of Radioactive Material in Controlled Areas. No user shall posses radioactive material in such a manner as to cause any individual in a controlled area to be present in an airborne concentration of radioactive material which, when averaged over 40 hours in any week, exceeds the limits specified in: (1) Section 30355, Appendix A, Table I, if the individual is 18 years of age or over; or (2) Section 30355, Appendix A, Table II, if the individual is under 18 years of age.

30277.   Bio-Assays and Medical Surcillance. (a) Each user shall make provision for a regular bio-assay program where indicated by and appropriate to the nature of potential exposure. (b) Each user shall make provision for review by a qualified physician of cases of known or suspented exposure exceeding permissible values and, as deemed necessary by said physician, medical examination, including tests and analyses where indicated, and treatment.

C. 10 CFR 20

20.101 Exposure of individuals to radiation in restricted areas.

(a) Except as provided in paragraph (b) of this section, no licensee shall possess, use, or transfer licensed material in such a manner as to cause any individual in a restricted area to receive in any period of one calendar quarter from radioactive material and other sources of radiation in the licensee's possession a dose in excess of the limits specified in the following table:

Rems per calendar quarter	
1. Whole body; head and trunk; active blood-forming organs; lens of eyes: or gonads	1 1/4
2. Hands and forearms; feet and ankles . . .	18 3/4
3. Skin of whole body	7 1/2

(b) A licensee may permit an individual in a restricted area to receive a dose to the whole body greater than that permitted under paragraph (a) of this section, provided:

(1) During any calendar quarter the dose to the whole body from radioactive material and other sources of radiation in the licensee's possession shall not exceed 3 rems; and

(2) The dose to the whole body, when added to the accumulated occupational dose to the whole

body, shall not exceed 5 (N—18) rems where "N" equals the individuals age in years at his last birthday; and

(3) The licensee has determined the individuals accumulated occupational dose to the whole body on Form AEC-4, or on a clear and legible record containing all the information required in that form; and has otherwise complied with the requirements of 20.102. As used in paragraph (b), "Dose to the whole body" shall be deemed to include any dose to the whole body, gonads, active bloodforming organs, head and trunk, or lens of eye.

20.103 Exposure of individuals to concentrations of radioactive material in restricted areas.

(a) No licensee shall possess, use or transfer licensed material in such a manner as to cause any individual in a restricted area to be exposed to airborne radioactive material possessed by the licensee in an average concentration in excess of the limits specified in Appendix B, Table I, of this part. "Expose" as used in this section means that the individual is present in an airborne concentration. No allowance shall be made for the use of protective clothing or equipment, or particle size, except as authorized by the Commission pursuant to paragraph (c) of this section.

(b) The limits given in Appendix B, Table I, of this part are based upon exposure to the concentrations specified for forty hours in any period of seven consecutive days. In any such period where the number of hours of exposure is less than forty, the limits specified in the table may be increased proportionately. In any such period where the number of hours of exposure is greater than forty, the limits specified in the table shall be decreased proportionately.

(c) (1) Except as authorized by the Commission pursuant to this paragraph no allowance shall be made for particle size or the use of protective clothing or equipment in determining whether an individual is exposed to an airborne concentration in excess of the limits specified in Appendix B, Table I.

(2) The Commission may authorize a licensee to expose an individual in a restricted area to airborne concentrations in excess of the limits specified in Appendix B, Table I, upon receipt of an application demonstrating that the concentration is composed in whole or in part of particles of such size that such particles are not respirable; and that the individual will not inhale the concentrations in excess of the limits established in Appendix B, Table I. Each application under this subparagraph shall include an analysis of particle sizes in the concentrations; and a description of the methods used in determining the particle sizes.

(3) The Commission may authorize a licensee to expose an individual in a restricted area to airborne concentrations in excess of the limits specified in Appendix B, Table I, upon receipt of an application demonstrating that the individual will wear appropriate protective equipment and that the individual will not inhale, ingest or absorb quantities of radioactive material in excess of those which might otherwise be permitted under this part for employees in restricted areas during a 40-hour week. Each application under this subparagraph shall contain the following information:

(i) A description of the protective equipment to be employed, including the efficiency of the equipment for the material involved;

(ii) Procedures for the fitting, maintenance and cleaning of the protective equipment; and

(iii) Procedures governing the use of the protective equipment, including supervisory procedures and length of time the equipment will be used by the individuals in each work week. The proposed periods for use of the equipment by any individual should not be of such duration as would discourage observance by the individual of the proposed procedures; and

(iv) The average concentrations present in the areas occupied by employees.

20.108 Orders requiring furnishing of bio-assay services.

Where necessary or desirable in order to aid in determining the extent of an individual's exposure to concentrations of radioactive material, the Commission may incorporate appropriate provisions in any license, directing the licensee to make available to the individual appropriate bio-assay services and to furnish a copy of the reports of such services to the Commission.

APPENDIX B

Definitons (Units in parenthesis)

Bioassay
The measurement, either direct or indirect, of the amount of radioactive material in the human body.

Body Burden
The quantity of radioactive material in the whole human body (μCi).

Dose Commitment
The internal dose equivalent resulting from an internal exposure (rem). Same as internal dose and internal dose equivalent.

40 MPC-hours
A term describing a personnel exposure to concentrations of radioactive material. An exposure of 40 MPC-hours is that which would result from being exposed to one MPC for 40 hours or 40 x MPC for one hour, etc. (μCi-hrs per cc).

Internal Absorbed Dose
The quotient of the energy imparted by internal ionizing radiation to the matter in a volume element with a given mass (rad).

Internal Dose
Same as internal absorbed dose.

Internal Dose Equivalent (I. D. E.)
The quantity obtained by weighting the internal absorbed dose by appropriate factors (rem) the I. D. E. is numerically equal to the internal absorbed dose in rad multiplied by the quality factor and any other modifying factors recommended by the ICRP.

Internal Dosimetry

The total process of measuring and calculating internal dose equivalent.

Internal Exposure

The quantity of radioactive material in the body or an organ of the body for a specified period of time (μCi-days). It is numerically equal to the time integral of the quantity of radioactive material in the body or organ (from time of exposure to infinity).

Internal Monitoring

The program of actions which results in determination of internal exposure.

Internal Ionizing Radiation

Radiation originating from an internal exposure consisting of charged particles (electrons, protons, alpha-particles, etc.) having sufficient kinetic energy to produce ionization by collision or uncharged particles (neutrons, photons, etc.) which can liberate charged particles or can initiate a nuclear transformation.

Maximum Permissible Body Burden

The quantity of radioactive material in the whole body which, if maintained, will result in the maximum permissible dose equivalent to the critical organ (μ Ci).

MPC-year

A term describing a personnel exposure to concentrations of radioactive material (μCi-years/cc). An exposure of one MPC-year is that which would result from being exposed to one MPC for one year, 12 times MPC for one month, 52 times MPC for one week, etc. One MPC-year results in the PAMDO.

Maximum Permissible Organ Burden

The quantity of radioactive material in an organ which will result in the maximum permissible internal dose (μCi).

Organ Burden

The quantity of radioactive material in an organ of the human body (μCi).

Permissible Annual Maximum Dose Commitment (PAMDO)

Dose equivalent resulting from a body intake of a radionuclide by a person occupationally exposed for one year at the maximum permissible concentration of that radionuclide (rem/year).

LICENSURE OF RADIOBIOASSAY
LABORATORIES

J. E. Regnier, A. A. Moghissi, R. T. Moore*
Southeastern Radiological Health Laboratory
Montgomery, Alabama

INTRODUCTION

In December of 1967 the Clinical Laboratories Improvement Act of 1967 was passed by the United States Congress. The purpose of this Act is to provide for the regulation and licensure of laboratories which accept for analysis specimens taken from the human body and transported in interstate commerce, provided that these specimens are taken for the "purpose of providing information for the diagnosis, prevention or treatment of any disease or impairment of, or the assessment of the health of man."**

---

*Bureau of Radiological Health; Rockville, Maryland.
**Quotation taken from Federal Register Title 42 Part 74. Unless otherwise noted, additional quotations in the paper are from this source or Clinical Laboratories Improvement Act of 1967.

It is of interest to health physicists that two types of
radiological laboratories come under the jurisdiction of
this Act: those laboratories which analyze specimens for
the purpose of assessing body concentrations of radionuclides—termed radiobioanalytical laboratories; and
those laboratories which perform procedures utilizing
radionuclides as tracers in their analytical procedures—
termed clinical radiochemistry laboratories. For purposes of the Act these two types of laboratories are
classified as radiobioassay laboratories.

The purpose of this paper is to describe the proposed implementation of the Act as it is applied to these
radiobioassay laboratories.

ADMINISTRATION

The responsibility for the Act has been given to
the Secretary of the Department of Health, Education,
and Welfare and is further delegated to the Director,
National Communicable Disease Center (NCDC), U.S.
Public Health Service, for implementation. To carry
out those provisions applying to radiobioassay laboratories, the Bureau of Radiological Health and specifically the Southeastern Radiological Health Laboratory
(SERHL) have provided consultative services to the
NCDC.

In addition to the aforementioned federal responsibilities, the Act provides that accreditation of laboratories by applicable state laws or by other accreditation
bodies may be accepted by the Secretary in lieu of
federal licensure. The criteria for such exemption are
that the standards applied by the accrediting agency are
equal to or more stringent than the provisions of the

Act and the rules and regulations issued pursuant to it. These standards must be reviewed by the Secretary at least annually, but more frequently if deemed necessary by the Secretary.

ESSENTIAL ELEMENTS

The Act and the regulations pertaining to it have four essential elements defining those areas for which licensure criteria are developed and which will be the basis for implementation of the Act. These are:

(i) maintenance of a quality control program adequate and appropriate for accuracy of the laboratory procedures and services;

(ii) maintenance of records, equipment, and facilities necessary to proper and effective operation of the laboratory;

(iii) qualifications of the director of the laboratory and other supervisory professional personnel necessary for adequate and effective professional supervision of the operation of the laboratory (which shall include criteria relating to the extent to which training and experience shall be substituted for education); and

(iv) participation in a proficiency testing program established by the Secretary.

Compliance with standards applicable to the first three of these areas will be determined by application review and on-site inspections. Assessment of compliance with the proficiency testing requirements will be based on data developed by each laboratory through participation

in an established proficiency testing program. The
following paragraphs describe the proposed standards
for (i) through (iv) and their intended application to
those laboratories involved in radiobioassay.

Quality Control

The basic intent of quality control criteria is to
ensure that, in addition to the reliability of the chemical procedures, radioactivity counting equipment is
functioning properly while in use. Within this premise,
all such equipment will be monitored each day of use
for critical operating characteristics. As an approximate evaluation of the proper functioning of the equipment with respect to these characteristics and as a
measure of the stability of the instrumentation, radioactive performance standards or reference sources
shall be counted at least once on each day of use. As
a more exact evaluation of the equipment operation as
well as associated chemical procedures, reference calibration samples containing known amounts of activity
and within expected levels of normal samples shall be
processed in replicate at least quarterly. Appropriate
records documenting each of the aforementioned determinations shall be maintained and be available to the
staff and to the Secretary.

Personnel Standards

The regulations of the Act prescribe standards for
the qualifications of the director and supervisor of
laboratory operations. Depending on the magnitude of
the operation, the director and supervisor may be the
same individual. The qualifications of these individuals

determine the categories in which a laboratory may be licensed. The aforementioned qualifications are generally based on those developed for administration of the program, Federal Health Insurance for the Aged. These are published in the Code of Federal Register Title 20, Chapter III, Part 405.

The standards prescribe academic and experience requirements for each category of laboratory analysis. For those personnel who do not meet these requirements an exemption is provided if they were directing or supervising a laboratory for 12 months in the 5-year period preceding July 1, 1966, and can pass an appropriate U. S. Public Health Service examination. For the category of radiobioassay, such an examination has not yet been developed.

For radiobioassay, the standards proposed are that the director or supervisor shall be a physician or shall hold an earned doctoral or master's degree in the chemical, physical, or biological sciences from an accredited institution and subsequent to graduation shall have had at least one year of experience in radiobioassay.

Proficiency Testing

The proficiency testing program of the Act is designed to provide a system for comparison of the analytical capability of regulated laboratories with other regulated laboratories and with reference laboratories having established competence.

Initial standards have been developed with the realization that few data are available on the accuracy and precision obtainable with a majority of the methods used in radiobioassay. Thus, these initial standards are relatively unrestrictive and as experience is gained, it may be necessary and desirable to make them more stringent.

In the conduct of the program, the aforementioned reference laboratories will be requested to perform their analyses by the most accurate method possible regardless of the time required. Thus, their results will be utilized to establish the true or target composition of the sample and the lowest practical standard deviation for an analysis.

For radiobioassay laboratories, a proficiency testing result will be acceptable if it falls within the central 95% of all laboratories, provided that no result will be unsatisfactory if it falls within the lowest and highest result obtained by the reference laboratories.

For both applicant and reference laboratories a result may be discarded if obviously deviant, provided that no more than 5% of the total results can thus be rejected.

Initial proficiency testing of radiobioassay laboratories will concentrate on those analyses most commonly performed. For radiobioanalysis these procedures will include urinalysis such as for ^{3}H and ^{90}Sr and for clinical chemistry the T-3 and T-4 tests of thyroid function.

Records

The Act provides for maintenance of records on samples received, analyses performed, and personnel directing, supervising and conducting the analyses. These records must be maintained for at least two years and be available on request for inspection.

SIGNIFICANCE OF ACT TO HEALTH PHYSICISTS

Successful implementation of the Act will help to ensure that health physicists are consistently provided with accurate personnel exposure data.   In addition, however, it should also be a valuable source of information on the accuracy, prevision, and reliability of various analytical methods.

A less direct, but no less important aspect is the legislative recognition of the health physics field in general and radiobioassay in particular.   Such recognition may serve as an impetus for accelerated refinement and new development of efficient, accurate and inexpensive bioassay techniques.

STATE RESPONSIBILITIES IN ESTABLISHING OFF-SITE EMERGENCY PLANS FOR NUCLEAR POWER REACTORS

James E. Martin
U. S. Public Health Service
National Center for Radioligical Health
Rockville, Maryland

INTRODUCTION

Public health agency programs involving the nuclear power industry must include adequate planning for responding to uncontrolled releases of radioactivity whether it occurs as a result of a small incident or the unlikely event of a major accident. Failure to do so may require the public to assume an unnecessary risk. Unfair criticism of the nuclear power industry as being grossly unsafe may also result. The operator of the facility may be forced to take the full brunt of the blame for public damage when, in fact, the fault may partially be due to poor planning. The health agency and the power company should therefore work jointly to develop plans to detect, evaluate, and limit the consequences of a complete spectrum of uncontrolled releases of radioactivity to the environment.

1825

The Nuclear Facilities Branch of the Division of
Environmental Radiation, Bureau of Radiological
Health, for several years has encouraged states to
work with the operators of nuclear power plants in the
cooperative development of radiological response plans
for possible incidents involving these facilities. In
this endeavor, we are now working with four states
that have power reactors in or near operation. Nine
states have reactors within 24 months of operation,
and emergency planning discussions are being held.
We have worked extensively with only one state at the
construction permit stage, but planning at this stage
is expected to increase since many power companies
are now providing more information on emergency
planning in Preliminary Safety Analysis Reports which
are submitted to the Atomic Energy Commission in
support of their application for a construction permit
and operating license.
    The discussion that follows is a summary of
factors learned in this work with states.

PLANNING CONSIDERATIONS

Among the major reasons for protective action
planning are the following:

1. Although the probability of an accident is low,
    the consequences could be severe.

2. The increased numbers of power reactors
    presently being planned or built may increase
    the probability of incidents or accidents oc-
    curring.

3. The current trend toward higher power levels will result in a greater accumulation of fission products and, therefore, an increase in the potential hazard.

4. Economic factors in power distribution are tending to bring reactor sites in closer proximity to population centers with a resultant increase in the projected consequences of an accident.

Each of these factors concerns the State health agency for a very basic reason: Once radioactivity is released to the off-site environs, it becomes the responsibility of the State health agency to assess the impact on the public and to take actions to protect their health. It is recognized that the Atomic Energy Commission issues a license to construct and operate the facility based on reasonable assurance that the safety and welfare of the public will not be jeopardized. However, it's authority to initiate protective actions is not clearly defined in the event of an accident, where areas outside the facility site are affected unless it is on behalf of the State or local government and with its permission. Within this context, when protective action is required to reduce the availability of radionuclides to the public in food products, such as milk, only the State has authority to act.

In addition to its licensing authority, the Atomic Energy Commission administers the provisions of Title 10 Part 140 of the Code of Federal Regulations which established financial protection requirements as contained in the Price-Anderson Indemnity Act. This Act provides for financial reimbursement for liability claims resulting from a nuclear facility accident.

Recent amendments to these Regulations provide for
prompt compensation from the hazardous properties
of radioactive material in the event of an extraordinary
nuclear occurrence and establish criteria by which
the AEC can determine whether or not such an event
has occurred in order that prompt payment can be
made to claimants.

The AEC has developed an assistance plan in
cooperation with other Federal and State agencies,
but this plan provides advice and assistance in public
health matters only at the request of the proper State
or local authority. For this reason, health agencies
must assume leadership in developing emergency
plans for radioactivity released to public areas.

Not only must they assume leadership in pro-
posing a plan but they must act efficiently and with
authority in executing it. Liaison should be established
with the power company prior to construction of a
nuclear power plant and should continue throughout
plant operation.

Although planning is usually initiated based on the
major accident, it is just as important to consider
smaller incidents which are more likely to occur.
These incidents are less likely to be reported quickly,
thus close cooperation, agreed upon in advance, is
necessary between the power company and the health
agency. Because of problems such as this, it is
imperative that written plans be developed that detail explicitly areas of responsibility, authority to
act, available resources, trained personnel, and
notification criteria. A general plan is desirable to
outline the parties involved and their responsibilities;
plans that specify detailed procedures for each parti-
cipant should be appended to the general plan. It is

also advisable to obtain written agreement on the plan to make it binding on the parties involved.

A major reactor accident is relatively easy to identify and conservative protective actions can be justifiably taken. Although the appropriate action may not be readily apparent in some cases, there is no question that notification of health and regulatory officials is necessary and that action must be taken. This distinction is more difficult, however, for the wide spectrum of incidents which could occur ranging from any release above normal operating levels up to a major contaminating event. In this broad range, guidance must be developed for notification criteria, for methods of evaluating the release, for initiation of protective action, and the appropriate decision basis. The Bureau of Radiological Health is currently studying this broad spectrum of incidents and the guidance required in order to determine what program efforts are needed to better define the problem in this area.

PLAN DEVELOPMENT

During development of protective action plans, the health agency should evaluate resources available for emergencies including police, radiation monitoring capabilities, communications, medical facilities, transportation, and radiological laboratory capabilities. Detailed plans should contain: 1) a clear understanding of responsibility and authority to act in the event of an accident; 2) criteria that require notification of health and regulatory agencies; 3) a list of personnel to be contacted and phone numbers; 4) provision for sufficient instrumentation, both on-site and

off-site, to detect an emergency condition quickly and
to determine the extent of contamination; 5) guidelines
for implementation of protective actions to limit the
spread of contamination and minimize the radiation
dose delivered to the public; 6) considerations for decontaminating, moving, and providing adequate medical
care for injured people; 7) guidelines for determining
if evacuation of the public is required and evacuation
procedures; 8) periodic tests of monitoring systems
to determine if they will function under accident conditions; and 9) periodic testing of the plan to assure
up-to-date competence in its execution.

One of the most important aspects of emergency
planning a State should consider is the availability of
resources to augment its own plan. The Interagency
Radiological Assistance Plan (IRAP) participants
which include among others the Atomic Energy Commission and the Public Health Service, can make
available the resources of their laboratories and technical personnel, organized into assistance teams, for
responding to nuclear accidents of any type.

The Bureau of Radiological Health also provides
assistance to State health agencies in protective action
planning for radiological emergencies in addition to its
IRAP participation responsibilities. The states are
encouraged to have specific plans for each nuclear
power plant in the state that can be integrated with a
statewide radiological response plan. Guidance is
provided on methods of evaluating the incident, protective actions that should be taken, and the basic
considerations that go into decisions to take these
actions. This role is important in providing uniformity
in state emergency planning. This becomes particularly important when a reactor is located where an

accident could release radioactivity into two or more
states. In these situations interstate agreements are
recommended.

PROBLEM AREAS

In some cases the role of the state and its authority and responsibilities with regard to nuclear power
plant incidents is not completely understood by either
state agencies or facility operators. This is evident
in some states where emergency plans for nuclear
power facilities in operation are not cooperative documents between the state and the power company, but
exist in the facility operating manual, a condition required by the Atomic Energy Commission for an operating license. There is little evidence that existing facility operation plans were developed cooperatively with
state agencies where the potential contamination of
off-site areas is a consideration. The role of the
State as a dynamic party in response to nuclear facility
incidents must be clearly recognized.

The lack of active state leadership in an area that
is logically part of its responsibility to the public is
partly due to the prevalent misunderstanding of the
respective authorities and responsibilities of the State
and Federal agencies. The Bureau of Radiological
Health has attempted, in its traditional advisory role,
to inform the states and the utilities of the need for
close cooperation in the establishment of emergency
plan agreements. In several states where recommendations on emergency planning for reactors have been
made by the Bureau of Radiological Health, state personnel expressed the belief that authority and

responsibility for action to protect the public in off-
site areas in the event of nuclear plant accidents was
that of the Atomic Energy Commission rather than
the state. We know of no instance where the AEC
has made such a determination. The Interagency
Radiological Assistance Plan alludes to state responsibility and authority relative to that of Federal
agencies, but clearer understanding in this area would
be helpful. An example of recognition of state authority was provided by the Advisory Committee on Reactor
Safeguards (ACRS) in its report on the Pilgrim Station
in Massachusetts. The ACRS recommended that the
operator of the proposed plant assure itself that the
state would be able to meet its responsibility in emergencies. This lack of understanding of state responsibility and authority is a problem area that must be
resolved in order to effectively plan for reactor incidents affecting the public. Considerable progress has
been made in this area and, hopefully, the situation
will continue to improve.

A second problem area involves notification criteria. Most power companies understandably are
reluctant to risk unnecessary public alarm by calling
public agencies before they have clear information
concerning what happended or for incidents that have
apparently caused no release. Unfortunately this re-
luctance can deprive the state of valuable time in
assessing the incident. Most states with which we
have worked don't desire immediate notification for
anything that is routine, but most certainly want to
know about incidents which have the potential to produce significent off-site releases of radioactivity. Power companies seem to fear exaggerated reports regarding
an incident which might create unfavorable publicity.

This fear is often justified in cases where plans are written principally for the major reactor accidents. Plans should have graded response levels including provisions for small incidents that require no more than an awareness by the State with confirmation either by plant data or a minimum of environmental samples taken under routine conditions. Developing mutual trust and respect is the logical approach for a state and a reactor plant operator to take in eliminating this problem. Plant conditions as well as radiation discharge levels should be considered in the notification criteria.

One state with which we have worked recently in developing an emergency plan for a facility has preferred to specify the same notification criteria for a nuclear facility as that stated in its state radiation code. These criteria are basically discharge levels specified by the Code of Federal Regulations, Title 10, Part 20 (10CFR20) Sections 20.403 and 20.405. Notification of smaller incidents is being attempted by a close working relationship (not formally written) with the power company. Another state, however, has been more stringent requiring notification with specific data from the reactor control room.

A third problem area involves protective actions and the decision basis for initiating them. Most planning emphasizes the use of general kits with portable instrumentation to make measurements. For example, one of the purposes for these measurements would be to obtain data upon which decisions could be made by competent authority for evacuation of public areas. None of the states with which we have worked have established guidelines for protective actions, and it appears that such guidance is needed. Population

density is an example of an important parameter requiring consideration in the development of these
guidelines. There is little understanding of the mean-
ing of exposure-rate measurements that would be
taken downwind of reactor accidents in terms of projected population dose. Considerable study is required to specify the various nuclides that would be
released, their percentages of total composition, deposited amounts, and the dose-rate and decay rate of
the deposited nuclides so that total integrated doses
can be reasonably estimated. Although guidance by
the Federal Radiation Council is available on protective action measures, additional guidance on
critical radionuclides, specifically related to reactor
accidents would be most useful.

Protective actions relative to thyroid doses from
iodine in milk represent a significant problem. Protection of the public from this type of exposure is easily
achieved following a contaminating incident by removing cows from pasture or by diverting or condemn-
ing the milk, yet either action, especially the latter,
would attract unfavorable publicity. Unfavorably publicity associated with a food so critical for proper
nutrition is not desirable. However, condemnation
must be on the basis of health risk which must be determined by the health department. It is difficult to
know whether to allow some exposure or to divert
milk as soon as it is known that it will be contaminated.
This decision is especially difficult since affected
markets would probably be small and if the milk were
condemned any resulting shortage of milk could be replaced from other sources. Protective actions to
prevent even low doses may be justified; yet practical
or publicity considerations could influence less conservative action.

SUMMARY

The potential consequences of reactor accidents and the rapid growth in the number of facilities requires states to exercise their responsibility to protect the public by developing plans to resolve any incidents that might occur. Cooperative planning with the power companies is the best approach. Adequate notification criteria, equipment, methods, guidelines for protective actions, and outside resources should be defined and implemented in a dynamic fashion by the states. Cooperation, guidance, and assistance to states should be provided by the nuclear power industry, the Public Health Service, the Atomic Energy Commission, and the Federal Radiation Council to solve problem areas involving interpretation of authority and responsibility, establishment of notification criteria, and implementation of protective action measures.

INVESTIGATION OF RADIUM USE IN
AIRCRAFT INSTRUMENT DIAL COMPANIES

Jack C. Rogers,
Joseph E. Karbus
Radiological Health Division
Los Angeles County Health Department
Los Angeles, California

Since the discovery of radium by Marie Curie in 1898, its broad use in the fields of medicine and industry has proved largely to be a positive contribution to all mankind.

The value of radium as a medical tool was quickly identified, when in 1901 radium was used for treatment of certain tumors in Paris, just 3 short years after its initial discovery. The first application of radium in medical therapy interestingly enough, was in the form of an unsealed source in direct contact with the affected area and held in place with a dressing. The dangers of exposure from radium, unfortunately were not realized as quickly as its benefits and any historical recount of radiation deaths from improper use of radium will only be a rough estimate. It has been reported that in the first 40 years of this century about 2 lbs of radium were extracted from the earth's crust and that at least 100 people died from various misuses of this material.[1]

The best documented series of radium poisoning cases
revealed at least 41 workers in the radium dial painting
industry are known to have died as a result of poisoning.[2] It was the habit of the workers to tip the brushes
with their lips, thereby injecting some of the paint into
their bodies, causing eventual death.[3] A body burden
of from 2 to 10 micrograms of radium is usually fatal.[4]
Because of its unusual and potent properties, radium
was heralded by some as a pancea for many of man's
ills. Radium dissolved in water was sold by one company as a cure for everything from skin rash to syphilis.
After several people died from drinking this lethal concoction, advertising of this particular commodity was
eventually banned.[5] Other companies capitalized
through the sale of radium facial cream, tablets and
suppositories.[6] As recently as this decade, tourists
visiting the Radium Hotel in Espirito Santo, Brazil,
where high natural desposits of radioactive ores, including radium, are known to exist in the sandy shore-
lines, would choose to sit for hours in holes dug in the
sand where radioactive minerals were detected.[1] This
is considered by some tourists as a popular form of
health therapy.

One of the earliest uses of radium in industry was
as an activating agent in chemical luminous compounds
for instrument dials, watch dials, light switches, and
as foot traffic markers in blacked out ships during
World War II. Today, radium use is decreasing in all
areas because of the greater availability of less
hazardous radioactive materials and the smaller expense in utilizing the newer materials. In spite of this,
there is evidence of as many as 4500 facilities using
radium in some form throughout the United States.[7]
This number is equivalent to approximately half of

the total number of AEC licenses in existence in the United States, although there is still no control by any Federal Agency such as Atomic Energy Commission over the possession and use of radium. Some States such as California have instituted statewide radiological health programs which include licensing and surveillance of all radioactive materials both naturally occurring and manmade. The safe use of radium is one objective of this program and is based on good radium management with application of acceptable radiological health procedures. Accidents involving loss, overexposures and contamination are not uncommon with radium and continue to occur, many of which never come to the attention of responsible Federal, State or local agencies because licensing or registration is not required in many areas of the country.

Although cheaper and less hazardous radioisotopes are currently available as substitutes for many traditional applications of radium, it may be several generations before modern technology eliminates radium from its present significant role as a practical tool of medicine and industry.

When the City of Los Angeles radiation control program was extended in 1964 to the entire Country of Los Angeles, the Los Angeles County Health Department assumed a regulatory role in radiation control by contract with the California State Department of Public Health. Since radium, under California Law, became subject to the radiological safety standards of the State Code, a greater knowledge of the public use and misuse of radium immediately became available.

One area where significant observations were noted is in the use of radium by aircraft instrument

dial companies as a component of radioactive luminous paint. These companies usually obtained radium
luminous compound in the form of a powder, as a mixture of radium sulphate and zinc sulphide. This is
mixed with another medium to produce a thick paint
which is applied to a dial or pointer of an aircraft
instrument. From time to time, repair and/or
refinishing of luminescent surfaces is performed,
following removal of all or some of the old luminous
paint from the dial. The removal of old paint was
generally done beneath water or oil to inhibit airborne
dust particles with the liquid residue poured into the
sewer system. Paint removal was often a more
messy operation than the initial application of luminous
paint.

As a result of several investigations made by the
Radiological Health Division of the County Health Department in response to reported radiation hazards in
aircraft instrument repair companies, it was decided
that a comprehensive approach be made to determine
the nature and extent of the problem. An initial review of available records on instrument repair companies revealed 34 facilities were known to use or possess aircraft instruments and component parts such as
pointers and dials which contained radioactive luminescent paint. Subsequent research of public commercial
listings revealed a potential of several times this number who may be engaged in such activities in the
greater Los Angeles area. Visits were scheduled to
the 34 facilities to conduct a preliminary survey to
determine whether the use and handling of radioactive
dials constituted a radiation hazard sufficient to require licensing under the California Radiation Control
Regulations. When survey findings did not indicate

a need for licensing, special in house procedures
would be provided for handling radioactive instruments.
A copy of these procedures is attached as Exhibit "A".

The 34 facilities eventually visited included 2 large
commercial aircraft companies, 2 electric instrument
repair shops, 23 aircraft instrument repair shops and
7 small private aircraft companies.

A special form was prepared to aid the health physicist in making the preliminary survey and to establish
uniformity in the information obtained by each person.
It was hoped that this survey would provide certain
basic information relative to the quantity of radium on
hand, type of activity engaged in by the company and
extent of radiation levels and contamination.   A copy
of the survey form used is attached as Exhibit "B".

FINDINGS

1. Personnel

About 90 percent of the shops engaged in disassembly and repair operations where direct contact with
radioactive pointers and dials was involved, had restricted such routine functions to only one or two persons.   These technicians seldom had a work history of
more than 5 years because of the high turnover of
workers.   Other personnel performed functions of a
generally minor nature, such as receiving, storing
and shipping instruments, but were not considered to
have a likelihood of routine exposure to radiation.   A
bioassay program to determine radium content in the
body, such as whole body radium testing, will eventually become a condition of the radioactive material

EXHIBIT A

OFFICE OF COUNTY HEALTH DEPARTMENT

Radiological Health Division
625-3212, Ext. 281

PROCEDURAL GUIDE FOR HANDLING RADIOACTIVE INSTRUMENTS, DIALS
AND POINTERS IN AIRCRAFT INSTRUMENT REPAIR FACILITIES

1. Detect and identify radioactive instruments, dials and
    pointers. Use a suitable radiation detection instrument
    to check for radioactivity.

2. Confine disassembly repair and assembly to a specific
    area, with least possible traffic.

3. If instrument is disassembled, repaired or assembled,
    perform all handling on smooth non-porous easily
    cleanable bench surface. Floor surface must also be non-
    porous and easily cleaned.

4. Loose radioactive dials and/or pointers must be segre-
    gated and be placed in closed containers.

5. Dials and/or pointers shall be stored in a location and
    manner such that acceptable radiation levels are
    maintained. Posting shall be in accordance with the
    Regulations.

6. No smoking or eating is permitted in areas where radio-
    active parts are processed. Always wash hands with soap
    and water after handling radioactive parts.

7. Working surfaces must be cleaned after each daily
    operation involving handling of radioactive material.

8. Dials, pointers, stripping solution and/or residue no
    longer useable must be transferred to a radioactive
    materials licensee authorized to receive such material.

JEK:lp
11/20/68

EXHIBIT B

Exhibit "B"

RADIUM SURVEY - AIRCRAFT INSTRUMENT REPAIR FACILITIES
Radiological Health Division
Los Angeles County Health Department

Name _____   Phone _____

Address _____

Owner _____   Phone _____

Persons Contacted _____   Date _____   Investigator _____

1. Number of Employees _____ (total)

    a. Handling unsealed Radium _____   Under 18 _____

2. Radium Inventory

    a. Instruments _____   Estimated Curiage _____

    b. Dials only _____   Estimated Curiage _____

    c. Handling & Repairing/mc _____   Estimated Curiage _____

    Stripping or refinishing _____   Describe under "Remarks". If no - complete below

        Stripping done by _____

        _____

3. Designated Area for Radium _____

4. Survey Instruments _____

5. Safety Procedures _____

6. Survey - External Levels   Contamination
    mr/hr   Location   mr/hr   Location

7. Remarks _____

T-137 (8/68)

license to be issued to those facilities required to get
such license.

2. Inventory of Radioactive Instruments

The number of radioactive aircraft instruments
on hand varied from none to approximately 5,000. The
presence of radioactive material on these instruments
was identified with a 1.4 mg/cm^2 Pancake Probe Geiger
Counter. These large inventories of instruments were
built up over a period of many years to provide a stock
of replacement parts. Generally, these items were
stored on open shelves inside of the facility, but in a
few instances were stored uncovered and uncontrolled
on open lots outside the building. A similar accumulation of loose radioactive dials and pointers were found
that had been removed from instruments cannibalized
for replacement parts. Quantities up to as many as
3000 individual pointers and dials were on hand at a
given facility, and were stored in paper bags, cigar
boxes or kept loose in drawers or on shelves throughout the facility. The concentration of such items in
large quantities was found to produce external radiation
levels as high as 30 milliroentgens per hour (mR/hr)
in the center of a workroom. Since many pointers and
dials were quite old, there was a tendency for the dried
luminous compound to flake off producing radioactive
contamination wherever they were stored.

Estimates of the amount of radium activity present
were made from rough gamma measurements with a
geiger counter. A number of representative dials
and pointers checked indicated a range of activity from
as little as 1 microgram to as much as 100 micrograms of Radium 226 per pointer or dial. The average

activity of a single pointer or dial was estimated to be about 10 micrograms. Consequently, a facility possessing an inventory of roughly 5,000 radioactive instruments could have as much as 100 milligrams of Radium on the premises.

3. Nature of Activity

The type of activity conducted by the aircraft instrument repair facility could be classified in one or a combination of the following three basic categories:

1) Receipt and storage of complete intact aircraft instruments only.

2) Disassembly and repair of instruments only.

3) Stripping off old luminous paint from dials or pointers and refinishing with new luminous paint, either radioactive or non-radioactive.

4. External Radiation Levels

A Victoreen 440 Ion Chamber Survey Meter was used to measure external radiation levels at physically accessible points of occupancy by company workers. These levels varied widely from ambient background (less than 0.1 mR/hr to as much as 30 mR/hr in accessible work areas, but the majority of facilities did not exceed 2 mR/hr in any working area. It was later decided that those facilities with ambient radiation levels exceeding 2 mR/hr in any area accessible to workers must segregate and properly shield radiation sources to reduce external radiation to acceptable levels. A strong educational approach was considered necessary to accomplish this, especially in those cases where a license would not be issued for radium use.

5. Contamination

Surface wipes were taken with dry filter paper to determine the amount of removable radioactive contamination present on work surfaces and floors in working areas. These wipes were taken on dry absorbent Whatman 41 filter paper 1 1/2 inches diameter and measured for activity with a L-75D Landsverk Electrometer using a 0.005 microcurie bare radium source as a standard. The maximum contamination level found was 13,000 dpm for a 100 square centimeter surface area. This is over five times the recommended alpha level for an uncontrolled area.[8] Six of the facilities visited had levels ranging from 10,000 to 13,000 dpm/100 cm^2. The remainder of the facilities showed a wide spread of contamination levels varying between no detectable removable contamination up to 10,000 dpm per 100 square centimeters.

6. Radiation Safety Program

None of the facilities surveyed had established any form of radiation safety program designed to minimize potential radiation hazards and the attitude exhibited by management and workers alike was casual, at best. Approximately 25 per cent of the facilities visited were not aware that the instruments they possessed contained radioactive material in any form. In a relatively few instances, the quality of housekeeping evident was considered adequate to contain and control radiation exposure and contamination problems. Housekeeping was closely checked in those facilities where either instrument disassembly, repair, stripping or refinishing was performed and was rated either as good, average or poor. Good house-keeping is considered to be a facility with cleanable smooth surfaces throughout the work areas and evidence that the facility was cleaned routinely (daily) and all activities were handled in an orderly fashion. An average facility is one that had cleanable smooth working surfaces and showed evidence of only occasional cleaning (weekly or less). A poor facility was one that exhibited working surfaces that were neither cleanable or smooth or had evidence of excessive debris or dust present in the working areas. Eight facilities were considered to have good housekeeping, five facilities had average housekeeping and two were poor.

CONCLUSION

It can be seen that aircraft instruments or components derived therefrom such as pointers or dials previously made radioactive with radium luminous paint still can be found in commercial use in significant quantities. However, current specification requirements of the Federal Aviation Agency and Military Regulations no longer call for radium as the luminous material of choice. Further, the type of facility engaged in the use, repair or sale of these devices varies from War Surplus Stores to large commercial aircraft companies.

The survey of 34 facilities involved in this activity revealed that about 20 per cent of them have potential radiation exposure problems to personnel sufficient to require that they obtain a Radioactive Material License to insure proper radiological practices. This action is currently in process. None of the companies checked had evidence of any form of radiation safety control program except that some excellent physical housekeeping programs served remarkably well to inhibit production and spread of radioactive contamination.

REFERENCES

1. Merrill Eisenbud, Environmental Radioactivity, McGraw Hill, 1963, pp. 12 and 169.

2. Anonymous, Life Magazine, Vol. 31, No. 17, 1951, p. 18.

3. Frederick L. Hoffman, "Radium Neurosis", JAMA, Vol. 85, No. 13, Sept. 16, 1925, pp. 961-965.

4. Robley D. Evans, "Radium Poisoning", Monthly Labor Review, Vol. 28, No. 6, June 1929.

5. Anonymous, New York Times, April 1, 1932, p. 1, col. 2.

6. Denver Radium Service, Op. Cit.

7. John C. Villforth, "Problems of Radiation Control" Radium Hazards and Control, Vol. 79, No. 4, April, 1964.

8. M. J. Duggan, and B. E. Godfrey, "Some Factors Contributing to Internal Radiation Hazard in Radium Luminising Industry", Health Physics, Vol. 13, No. 6, June, 1967, p. 613.